HANDBOOK OF CANCER DIAGNOSIS AND STAGING
A Clinical Atlas

HANDBOOK OF CANCER DIAGNOSIS AND STAGING
A Clinical Atlas

Seth A. Borg, M.D.
Clinical Associate Professor of Radiology
University of Rochester School of Medicine
Consulting Radiologist
Department of Radiology
Division of Oncology
Rochester General Hospital
Rochester, New York

Susan Rosenthal, M.D.
Associate Professor of Oncology in Medicine
University of Rochester Cancer Center
Attending Physician
Department of Medicine
Division of Oncology
Rochester General Hospital
Rochester, New York

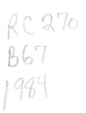
RC 270
B67
1984

A WILEY MEDICAL PUBLICATION
JOHN WILEY & SONS
New York • Chichester • Brisbane • Toronto • Singapore

Cover and interior design: Wanda Lubelska

Library of Congress Cataloging in Publication Data:

Borg, Seth A.
  Handbook of cancer diagnosis and staging.

  (A Wiley medical publication)
  Bibliography: p.
  Includes index.
  1. Cancer—Diagnosis—Handbooks, manuals, etc.
I. Rosenthal, Susan N.   II. Title.   III. Series.
[DNLM: 1. Neoplasms—Diagnosis.   2. Neoplasm staging.
QZ 241 B732c]
RC270.B67   1984   616.99′4075   83-14597
ISBN 0-471-87073-0

Printed in the United States of America

10 9 8 7 6 5 4 3 2 1

To our parents,
Esther and Harold Borg
and
Blanche and Robert Rosenthal,
with loving gratitude for their guidance
and unwavering encouragement through the years

FOREWORD

The successful management of patients with cancer requires a multidisciplinary team approach. Following the establishment of the tissue diagnosis of malignancy, the primary care physician (surgeon, family physician, or internist) has the responsibility to assess the extent of the disease, that is, whether it is localized, regional, or metastatic. The American Joint Commission has provided a detailed staging classification for each of the nonhemopoietic "solid tumors," using the "T" (tumor size), "N" (node status), and "M" (metastatic) system.

During the past decade there has been a virtual explosion in the development and installation of radiographic procedures to assist in the staging of patients with cancer. A variety of radionuclide studies (technetium-99m, gallium-67) with improved resolution of the scanners exist side by side with ultrasonography and constantly improving computerized axial tomography. In the near future, nuclear magnetic resonance (NMR), previously available only for radiobiologic research, will compete with CAT scanners. How does a physician choose among the options? Can he or she be expected to know the accuracy (i.e., sensitivity and specificity) of each test and, faced with escalating medical care costs in an era of apparent chronic recession, assess the cost effectiveness of the evaluation?

In this handbook Drs. Borg and Rosenthal have provided a succinct outline approach to these problems. Both are well qualified to address the issues raised. The text is brief and designed to provide an introduction to disease-specific staging. In addition to the chapters on radiographic evaluation and staging by tumor site, there are chapters dealing with two major oncologic problems: cancer of unknown origin and oncologic emergencies.

One of the unique aspects of this book is the excellent quality of the more than 100 black and white x-ray photographs that serve to illustrate the various stages of the neoplasms. In addition, a series of flow charts provides a step by step approach for the physician to follow in assessing his or her patients.

Finally, a few thoughts about the appeal of this handbook. Although the authors have designed the book primarily for medical students and generalists, the flow diagrams would serve very well instructors of oncology courses and directors of hematology/oncology training programs. Once staging is completed in the most cost-effective manner, then a therapeutic decision by a team of surgical, radiation, and medical oncologists can be made in the best interests of the patient.

John M. Bennett, M.D.
Professor of Oncology in Medicine
Head, Medical Oncology Division
University of Rochester Cancer Center
University of Rochester School of Medicine
 and Dentistry
Rochester, New York

PREFACE

The *Clinical Handbook of Cancer Diagnosis and Staging* was developed and written for primary care physicians and surgeons, house officers, and students as a guide to the diagnosis and subsequent staging of cancer. Recent and continuing advances in tumor imaging are presented, and the critical importance of cancer staging before initiating therapy is emphasized. Guidelines for evaluation of the major site-specific cancers are established on the basis of several principles: (1) efficient use of the current imaging armamentarium, (2) appropriate application of the information gained to clinical decision making, (3) avoidance of patient risk whenever possible, and (4) cost-effectiveness of the diagnostic process.

The conclusions reached are drawn from our clinical judgment and experience with hundreds of cancer patients. Our satisfaction in preparing this book will be complete if cancer patients receive more precise, thoughtful, and appropriate pretherapeutic evaluations.

Seth A. Borg
Susan Rosenthal

ACKNOWLEDGMENTS

With gratitude the authors wish to acknowledge the following people for their assistance and advice in the development of portions of this book: James C. Arseneau, M.D.; Mark Chodoff, M.D.; Laura vonDoenhoff, M.D.; Karin Dunnigan, M.D.; Philip Dvoretsky, M.D.; Raymond Gramiak, M.D.; J. Raymond Hinshaw, M.D.; Charles L. Lewis, M.D.; Eileen Paterson, M.D.; Robert J. Peartree, M.D.; Robert M. Spitzer, M.D.; Donald W. Spratt, M.D.; Robert S. Weiner, M.D.; and Paul E. Weiss, M.D. Special appreciation is due to Rochester Radiology Associates for their constant encouragement and support of this project.

Raymond A. Moloney of John Wiley & Sons provided invaluable editorial guidance from the germination of the concept to completion of the book. We are also indebted to Anita Matthews who produced the illustrations as well as to Cathleen Versage and Jane Stets who provided excellent secretarial support.

We are grateful to J.B. Lippincott Company for their generous permission to use the TNM and staging classifications for the various malignancies, and to the American Cancer Society for permission to use their 1983 cancer incidence statistics.

Seth A. Borg
Susan Rosenthal

CONTENTS

2
RADIOLOGIC EVALUATIONS BY SITE
61

3
DIAGNOSIS AND STAGING OF PRIMARY MALIGNANCIES
77

4

EVALUATION OF PATIENTS WITH CANCER OF UNKNOWN ORIGIN

5

ONCOLOGIC EMERGENCIES: DIAGNOSTIC EVALUATION

Introduction

The ultimate goal in the management of any patient with malignancy is curative treatment or, if this is not possible, improvement in the duration and quality of survival. While this may seem simplistic and self-evident, clinicians often lose sight of the ultimate objective while traveling through the maze of the diagnostic and staging evaluation. All too often patient needs are forgotten as diagnostic possibilities are pursued with relentless urgency using increasingly elaborate and esoteric tools. At times the diagnostic process seems to take on a momentum of its own, leaving patients and their problems far behind.

Thoughtful application of clinical and laboratory information can lead to a more rational and cost-effective evaluation of the cancer patient. Defining what information will be necessary for therapeutic decision making before embarking on an extensive laboratory and imaging work-up is more than just an academic exercise. Such definition may result in elimination of high-risk procedures, shorter hospital stays, and reduction in patient and family anxiety. Intelligent use of laboratory and clinical tools has far-reaching implications for treatment planning for the cancer patient.

Evaluation of the cancer patient begins with the clinical suspicion of malignancy (Figure I.1). Typically the patient presents to the primary physician with a complaint that immediately raises concern of possible malignancy. Common examples of such complaints include a history of rectal bleeding, the discovery of a breast lump, and a cough with hemoptysis. The physician's initial history and physical examination usually increase the suspicion of malignancy and result in a diagnostic suggestion of the presence of a malignant process. At this point consultations with specialists such as gastroenterologists, urologists, general surgeons, and medical imagers (radiologists) are frequently required. The primary physician, with the advice of his or her consultants, then plans the most expeditious method of obtaining histologic verification of malignancy. This represents a major undertaking in many cases and ideally requires a knowledge of all modalities that can be brought to bear on the particular clinical problem. In some instances a simple noninvasive procedure, such as sputum cytology, should be the initial approach, while in other cases computerized tomography or ultrasonography followed by percutaneous biopsy may be most appropriate. In other situations surgical exploration with open biopsy may prove the most expeditious first step. Selecting the verification technique should be a joint effort of the primary physician and consultants along with informed input and consent from the patient.

Following histologic verification of malignancy, treatment considerations

1

arise. Rarely can adequate treatment planning take place immediately following histologic diagnosis. In most cases the entire extent of the tumor must be assessed to allow an intelligent decision to be made from among the therapeutic options. Such an assessment requires an understanding of the typical pathways of spread for the particular malignancy under consideration.

Tumors spread primarily by three means: (1) direct extension by local invasion; (2) lymphatic extension; and (3) hematogenous dissemination.

Adequate evaluation of each of these compartments—tumor (T), node (N), and metastasis (M)—poses the next problem in the pretreatment evaluation of the cancer patient. Accurate knowledge of the extent of disease is essential for proper therapeutic decisions. Failure to evaluate disease extent fully can lead to tragic errors in management. For example, amputation of an extremity in a patient with osteogenic sarcoma without recognition of the presence of numerous pulmonary metastases would represent an entirely unnecessary and excessively radical treatment. Similarly, patients with metastatic carcinoma of the breast require a completely different approach from that employed for patients with disease limited to the breast. Also, a patient with a T1 NO-1 MO lung lesion may well be a surgical candidate. However, if the lesion is defined as T3, N2, or M1, most authorities would consider the patient incurable by surgery.

The TNM classification referred to above provides a standard terminology for describing disease extent in cancer patients. The TNM system brings some degree of uniformity and clarity to cancer staging, which in the past has been characterized by numerous conflicting and overlapping classifications, confusing to both specialists and generalists alike. Although not every tumor is amenable to TNM staging, this system should be used whenever possible and, where applicable, will be employed throughout this book.

With the use of an intelligent, thoughtful approach to tumor diagnosis and staging, and complete assessment of disease extent with description by the TNM classification (or other standard system for certain tumors), physicians will have the best opportunity to plan the optimal treatment for their patients with malignant disease. Treatment decisions based on adequate knowledge of tumor behavior and on hard, accurate evidence of tumor extent have the greatest chance of providing patient benefit while minimizing excessive risk and expense.

SCHEMA : Cancer Patient Evaluation

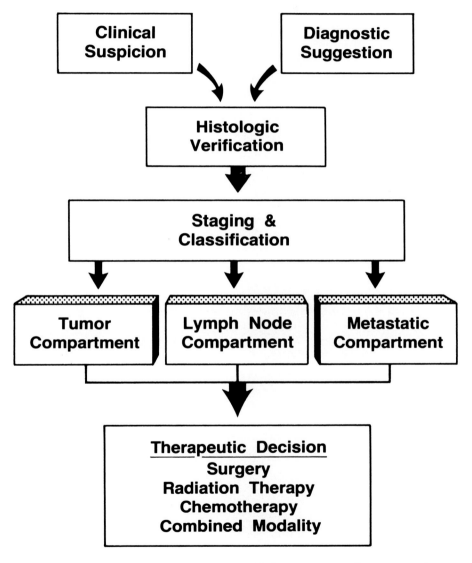

Figure 1.1 *Flow diagram for evaluation of the patient with suspected cancer.*

CHAPTER I

Imaging Modalities for Cancer Diagnosis and Staging

A thorough history and meticulous physical examination are still, as they were 50 years ago, the most important sources of diagnostic information for the physician. In the past half century, however, numerous high technology diagnostic procedures have been introduced, particularly in the area of medical imaging. Even newer modalities are not far off on the horizon. If physicians are to use these new procedures properly, they must understand how they are performed, what tests they replace, their risks and costs, and how they compare with similar investigations of the same anatomic site or organ system.

This chapter discusses each of these more sophisticated radiologic procedures, including practical details on how the examination is performed, what form of patient preparation is required, the risks of the procedure, and how it compares with other modalities that can be used to visualize the same area. A cost assessment is given in relative terms, with a single $ representing the least expensive examination and $$$$ indicating the most costly procedure.

Many of these procedures require the use of contrast media for optimal radiologic visualization. In many instances the contrast media themselves may produce certain side effects and complications, independent of the specific imaging procedure. While a complete review of radiologic contrast media is beyond the scope of this text, the most important untoward effects of such agents are outlined below.

RADIOLOGIC CONTRAST AGENTS

IODINATED WATER-SOLUBLE CONTRAST AGENTS

Iodinated water-soluble contrast agents, which are available under a wide variety of trade names, are used in urography, computerized tomography, angiography, venography, cholangiography, and other procedures of less relevance to the cancer patient. Untoward reactions to these agents occur in approximately 5% of patients examined. In the vast majority of cases the reactions are minor. The incidence of severe reactions is about 1 in 1000, and the overall death rate reported from intravascularly administered contrast media ranges from 1 in 10,000 to 1 in 40,000 examinations.

Minor reactions to iodinated water-soluble contrast agents include nausea and vomiting, pain in the arm, a sensation of generalized warmth or flushing, and a bitter taste in the mouth. No treatment is necessary, and the reactions subside promptly. Patients with a history of asthma, hay fever, urticaria, iodine sensitivity, and a previous reaction to a radiologic contrast agent have a greater incidence of subsequent reactions. Unfortunately, there is no way to predict whether a given patient will develop a reaction or not.

Side effects of intermediate severity are uncommon and include erythema, urticaria, asthma, and facial swelling. These reactions are not life-threatening, but they often require treatment such as injection of diphenhydramine or epinephrine for relief of symptoms.

Severe side effects—respiratory arrest, cardiac arrest, shock—require immediate emergency treatment. Fortunately such reactions are rare.

The pathophysiology of these reactions to iodinated water-soluble contrast agents is not well understood. Although a relationship between allergy and contrast reactions is clearly present, many authorities assert that allergic hypersensitivity represents only part of the problem. Anxiety, abnormal midbrain activity, and vascular injury have all been invoked as possible explanations of contrast reactions.

Patients with a history of previous reaction to a contrast agent can be restudied with an iodinated agent if the indication for the study is sufficient to make the risk acceptable, and if proper precautions are taken. Adequate equipment and personnel for cardiorespiratory resuscitation must be available and alerted. Prophylactic pretreatment with corticosteroids, antihistamines, and diazepam is advocated by some, but the efficacy of this prophylaxis has not been clearly demonstrated.

Deterioration in renal function is a predictable, preventable complication of the use of intravascular contrast media that has only recently been recognized. Particularly in hypotensive or dehydrated patients, patients with preexisting azotemia, and in multiple myeloma patients with Bence Jones proteinuria, intravascular contrast radiography may precipitate acute renal failure which in most cases is reversible. With adequate hydration before the examination, this complication can be avoided.

IODINATED INTRATHECAL CONTRAST AGENTS

Intrathecal contrast agents are employed in cancer patients in the study of the spinal subarachnoid space in cases of suspected spinal cord compression. Pantopaque, an oily contrast agent, may induce an irritative arachnoiditis and must be completely aspirated following myelography. Metrizamide, a water-soluble agent, does not appear to cause arachnoiditis and does not require aspiration. However, this agent may cause seizures in seizure-prone individuals if allowed to enter the cranium. Metrizamide offers the advantage of use in conjunction with computerized tomography of the spine, which allows highly detailed images of the vertebrae, spinal cord, and meninges to be obtained.

OILY CONTRAST AGENTS

In cancer patients oily contrast agents have their primary use in lymphography. The main complication here is due to the procedure rather than to the agent itself and consists of pulmonary microembolization of the contrast medium with resulting impairment of pulmonary function. This complication causes clinically significant toxicity only in patients with preexisting pulmonary dysfunction of moderate to severe degree.

BARIUM

Barium sulfate is a radiopaque nonabsorbable material employed in the study of the gastrointestinal tract. Complications do not arise unless perforation or obstruction is present. Spillage of barium into the peritoneal space may promote bacterial peritonitis. Impaction of ingested barium above a colonic obstruction may lead to additional morbidity.

7

ANGIOGRAPHY

ASSESSMENT

Before the advent of computerized tomography, angiography—the study of morphology based upon vascular appearance following contrast injection—offered the only means of detailed evaluation of tumor localization and extent. Although some imprecision became apparent as a result of surgical staging procedures and more sophisticated imaging techniques, angiography remained until recently the best tumor imaging modality available.

Currently, computerized tomography and ultrasonography have supplanted angiography in many situations. Nevertheless, angiography still has a crucial role when knowledge of the vascular anatomy of a tumor is essential prior to its attempted removal. Renal cell carcinomas, primary brain tumors, and pancreatic islet cell tumors, for example, are usefully studied with preoperative angiography.

INDICATIONS

1. Preoperative vascular mapping of certain primary tumors (Figure 1.1).
2. Localization of extremely small tumors, such as some pancreatic islet cell tumors.
3. Blood sampling of tumor effluent for certain tumor markers: that is, catecholamines elaborated by pheochromocytomas; parathyroid hormone by parathyroid tumors.

PREPARATION

1. Nothing by mouth (NPO) after midnight prior to the examination.
2. Assure adequate state of hydration.
3. Assure adequate renal function.
4. Check clotting parameters.

TECHNIQUE

After selection of an appropriate femoral artery (one with a good pulse), the overlying skin is prepared with surgical iodine, and the skin and soft tissues are infiltrated with local anesthetic. A percutaneous needle puncture of the artery (or vein if cavography is performed) precedes the insertion of a metallic guide wire, which is then threaded into the artery or vein. A catheter is passed over the guide wire and contrast is injected for assessment of the position of the catheter tip. Once proper position is achieved, a pressure injector is attached to the catheter, contrast is injected rapidly, and a series of x-rays is taken. Multiple "runs" (contrast injections followed by filming) may be taken with the patient in varying positions to obtain the best views of the area under study. Magnification views may be obtained resulting in highly detailed images.

Once the examination has been completed, the catheter is withdrawn and direct pressure is maintained over the arterial puncture site for 15 minutes to prevent bleeding. The patient then remains at bedrest without flexing the leg for the next several hours.

RISKS

1. Iodinated contrast reaction.
2. Local complications related to the arterial puncture, including thrombosis, distal embolization, and hemorrhage.

TIME REQUIRED

1–3 hours, depending on the anatomic area studied and technical factors.

COST

$$$

9

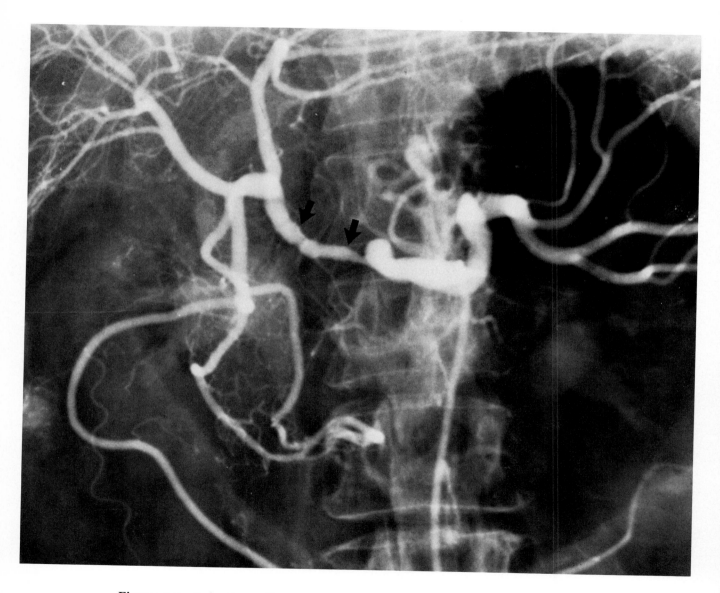

Figure 1.1 Selective celiac angiogram demonstrating encasement of the common hepatic artery (arrows) due to pancreatic carcinoma.

BARIUM
GASTROINTESTINAL STUDIES

ASSESSMENT

Over the past 50 years, the barium study has proved to be a safe and reliable tool for imaging the gastrointestinal tract. Barium study is the examination of choice for intraluminal visualization of the gastrointestinal tract. Double contrast examination, the combination of barium and air, permits radiologic visualization of very fine mucosal detail, and, for the detection of small cancers of the esophagus or the colon, double contrast study is ideal. Evaluation of extrinsic compression of the colon, small bowel, or esophagus, however, requires a coarser appraisal best served by barium alone.

INDICATIONS

1. Detection of primary malignancies of esophagus, stomach, small bowel, and large bowel (Figure 1.2).
2. Demonstration of gastrointestinal tract obstruction.
3. Evaluation of mediastinal adenopathy with a barium esophagram.

TECHNIQUE

Barium is ingested, injected through a nasogastric tube, or introduced into the colon by enema. Patient position is altered frequently during the examination to assure satisfactory coating of the intraluminal surfaces and to facilitate filling and emptying of specific areas such as the gastric fundus or the cecum.

Pharmacologic agents, such as glucagon, may be used to paralyze the motion of the stomach, duodenum, or colon temporarily, allowing very fine detail to be recorded on film.

PREPARATION

Esophagram: NPO after the midnight preceding the study. This will permit study of the stomach as well, if necessary.

Upper gastrointestinal series: NPO after midnight.

Barium enema: Requires scrupulous cleansing of the colon to eliminate confusing debris such as stool or mucus. Magnesium citrate, other laxatives, and tap water enemas are given the evening before the examination. On the morning

11

of the study additional enemas, given in the x-ray department just before the examination, are recommended.

RISKS

1. Aspiration in patients with esophageal obstruction.
2. Peritoneal contamination through a colonic or gastric perforation. (If a perforation is suspected, the examination should be performed with a water-soluble contrast agent.)
3. Although it is a misconception that barium can convert a partial to a complete small bowel obstruction, barium above a colonic obstruction may be converted to a hard concretion due to reabsorption of water by the colon. This can be avoided by examining suspected colonic obstructions from below (barium enema).

Cost:

$$

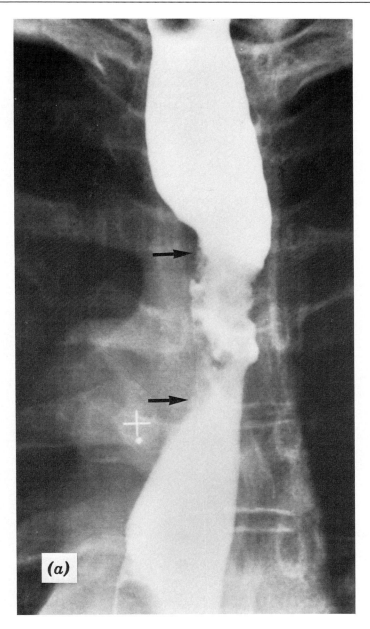

Figure 1.2 (a) Barium esophagram demonstrating circumferential primary esophageal carcinoma (arrows). (b) Barium enema of a patient with Burkitt's lymphoma. The terminal ileum (arrows) is deviated medially by a paracecal mass.

13

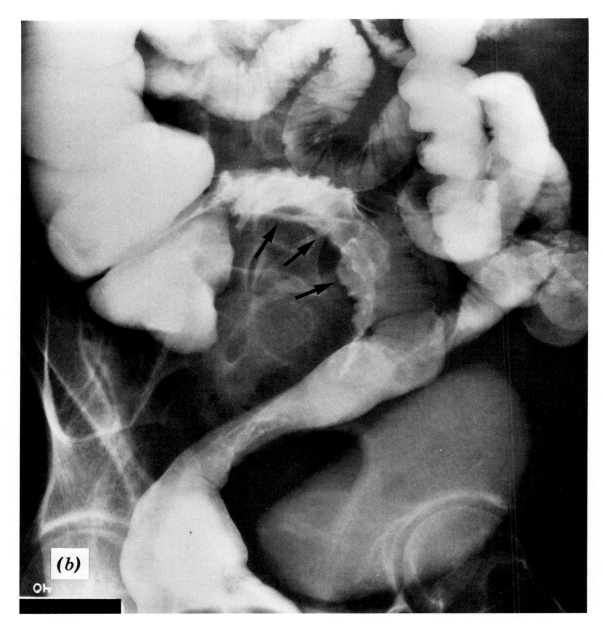

Figure 1.2 (Continued)

COMPUTERIZED TOMOGRAPHY

ASSESSMENT

Within the past few years computerized tomography (CT) has become the cornerstone of the diagnostic and staging assessment of most malignancies. In evaluating the primary tumor (T) itself, CT accurately depicts the size, location, and local extent of the lesion. The lymph node compartment (N), including mediastinal, retroperitoneal, and pelvic nodes, is readily visualized, although a negative CT study for adenopathy in many circumstances should be confirmed by surgical techniques.

In the assessment of suspected brain metastases, CT is the imaging modality of choice and has almost entirely supplanted radionuclide brain scanning and cerebral angiography for this indication. Benign lesions, including cerebral infarcts and abscesses, however, must be distinguished from metastatic deposits. Computerized tomography also provides highly sensitive and specific information in the evaluation of liver metastases.

INDICATIONS

1. Detection and evaluation of primary and metastatic malignancies (Figure 1.3).
2. Guidance for percutaneous biopsy procedures.

TECHNIQUE

The patient lies within a scanning gantry in which an x-ray tube and multiple x-ray detectors are located. The x-ray tube rotates about the patient taking multiple exposures. The information gathered by the detectors may be displayed in axial, sagittal, and coronal planes following computerized reconstruction.

In many cases the patient receives intravenous iodinated contrast to enhance the CT image. In the evaluation of spinal lesions a water-soluble myelographic contrast agent is often employed.

PREPARATION

1. NPO for several hours before the examination.
2. Eliminate any residual barium from previous gastrointestinal contrast examinations.
3. If intravenous contrast is used, assure adequate hydration and renal function.

RISKS

Iodinated contrast reaction.

TIME REQUIRED

30–60 minutes.

COST

$$$$

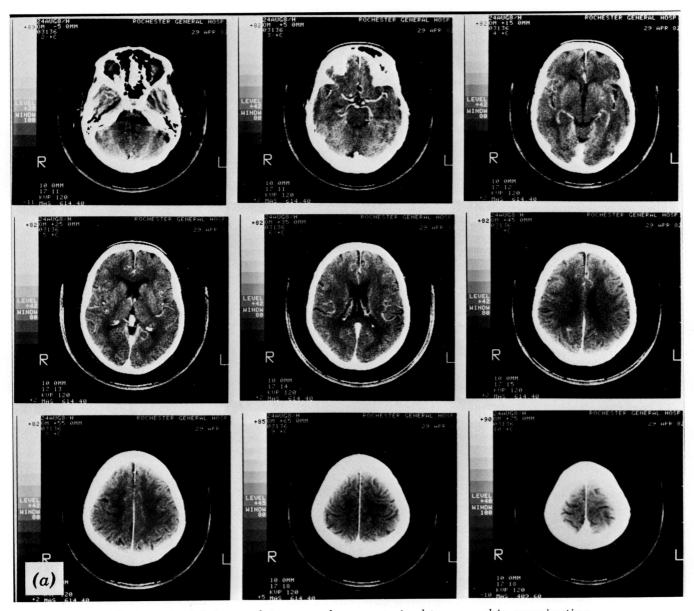

Figure 1.3 (a) A complete, normal, computerized tomographic examination of the head permitting visualization of the vessels in the circle of Willis by prior intravenous injection of iodinated contrast.

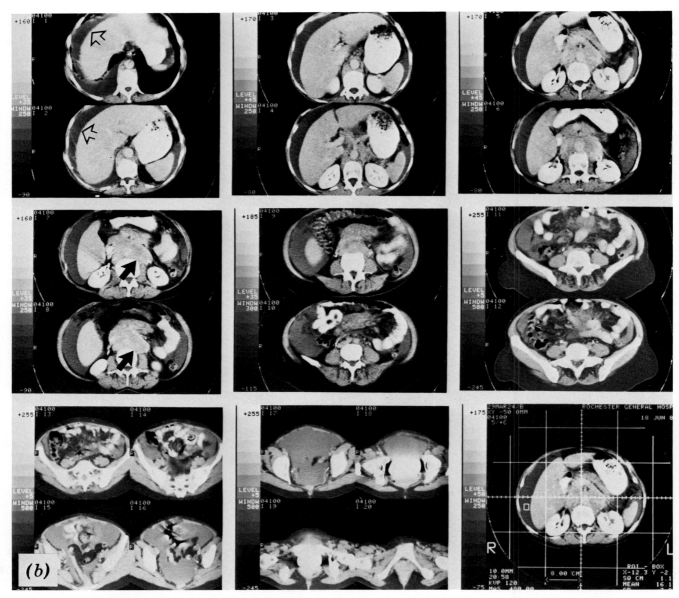

Figure 1.3 *(Continued) (b) A complete computerized tomographic study of the abdomen in a patient with ascites (open arrows, left image, top row) and para-aortic lymphadenopathy (solid arrows, left image, second row) due to non-Hodgkin's lymphoma.*

ENDOSCOPIC RETROGRADE CHOLANGIOPANCREAT- OGRAPHY

ASSESSMENT

Endoscopic retrograde cholangiopancreatography (ERCP) is an endoscopic procedure for evaluation of the pancreas and biliary system. The papilla of Vater is cannulated under direct vision, allowing injection of contrast into the pancreatic and common bile ducts. The procedure is successfully completed in about 90% of cases and is highly dependent on physician expertise.

In the evaluation of a pancreatic mass ERCP serves to delineate abnormalities in the pancreatic ductal system; these findings can be used to distinguish a neoplastic from an inflammatory process, which is often not possible by CT or ultrasonography. In addition, pancreatic duct fluids can be aspirated for cytologic analysis.

The common bile duct and some of its branches may also be visualized to evaluate obstruction in this area. Percutaneous transhepatic cholangiography (PTC) may offer greater definition of the type and location of the obstruction; however, ERCP offers an alternative in the patient with nondilated intrahepatic ducts or whose clotting function is abnormal, situations in which PTC may not be successful or is too risky.

INDICATIONS

1. Evaluation of a pancreatic mass: differentiation between a neoplastic and an inflammatory process.
2. Evaluation of biliary tract obstruction (Figure 1.4).

TECHNIQUE

Following adequate sedation of the patient and anesthesia of the oropharynx, a side-viewing fiberscope is passed through the mouth and into the duodenum. The papilla of Vater is identified and cannulated with a Teflon catheter. Water-soluble contrast is then injected through the cannula. As the ductal systems fill with contrast material, multiple x-ray films, in several views, are taken. The procedure can be done in an out-patient setting.

19

PREPARATION

1. NPO after midnight preceding the study.
2. Premedication with meperidine and atropine.
3. Prophylaxis with antibiotics if the biliary system is obstructed.
4. Anesthesia to the oropharynx with a topical agent.
5. Sedation with diazepam.
6. Intravenous glucagon to sustain duodenal ileus.

RISKS

1. Acute pancreatitis (usually mild) following injection of contrast.
2. Sepsis and abscess formation in previously existing pseudocyst.
3. Ascending cholangitis following injection of contrast into an obstructed common duct.

TIME REQUIRED

30–120 minutes.

COST

$$$$

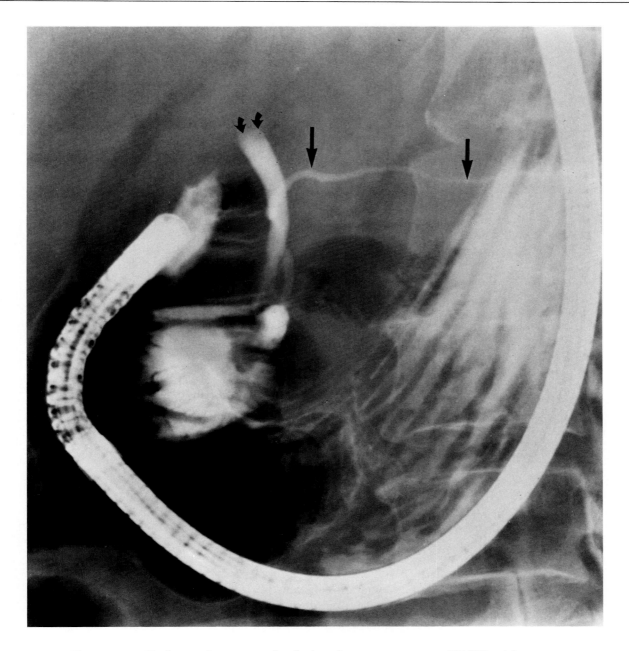

Figure 1.4 *Endoscopic retrograde cholangiopancreatogram (ERCP) with normal pancreatic duct (long arrows) and obstructed common duct at its midportion (short arrows).*

LYMPHOGRAPHY

ASSESSMENT

Before the introduction of computerized tomography and ultrasonography, lymphography was the only imaging tool allowing direct visualization of the abdominal lymph nodes. With the current availability of the two newer imaging modalities, however, the role of lymphography has become less clear. In general, when bulky lymph node disease is anticipated, as in the lymphomas, computerized tomography may be preferable. In such cases a negative CT scan is highly reliable. On the other hand, where lymph node involvement is not expected to cause increased nodal size, as in many solid tumors that destroy nodes, a negative CT scan is not as reliable. Therefore, for the staging of pelvic solid tumors, such as carcinomas of the bladder, cervix, and prostate, lymphography may be more useful. However, general agreement has not been reached as yet on the relative merits of CT, lymphography, and ultrasonography for pelvic and abdominal lymph node assessment.

INDICATIONS

1. Staging of pelvic cancers (prostate, testis, cervix, bladder, rectum).
2. Staging of Hodgkin's and non-Hodgkin's lymphomas (Figure 1.5).

TECHNIQUE

A blue dye is injected into the interdigital webs of the feet in order to demonstrate the lymphatic vessels. A surgical cut-down is then performed over a large dye-impregnated lymphatic, and the vessel is cannulated with a small needle. Contrast is injected slowly over a 1- to 2-hour period. After the contrast has filled the inguinal, iliac, and para-aortic lymph channels (lymphangiogram stage), x-ray films are taken in multiple projections. The patient is sent home over night but returns in 24 hours for additional films showing contrast present in lymph nodes (lymphadenogram or storage stage). In some centers an intravenous urogram is performed at the time of the 24-hour films.

PREPARATION

None. The patient must be able to lie still for about 2 hours while the injection is in progress.

RISKS

1. Idiosyncratic reaction to blue dye.
2. Iodinated contrast reaction.
3. Pulmonary dysfunction due to microembolization of the contrast medium (clinically significant only in patients with preexisting pulmonary impairment).

TIME REQUIRED

2–3 hours on day 1.
30 minutes on day 2 (60 minutes if urography performed).

COST

$$

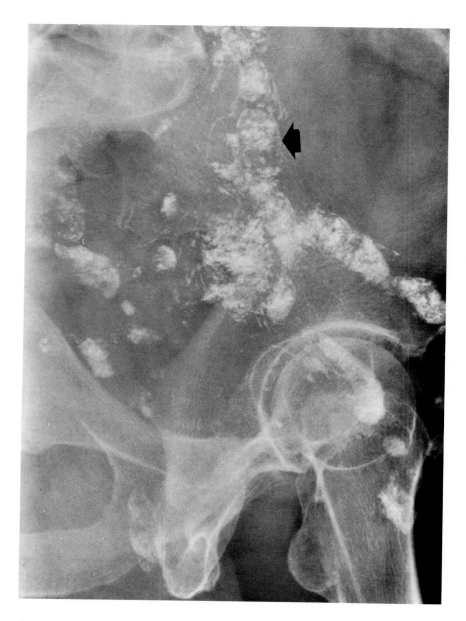

Figure 1.5 Lymphogram demonstrating severely distorted lymph nodes (arrow) partially replaced and enlarged by lymphoma.

24

MAMMOGRAPHY

ASSESSMENT

Current low-dose mammographic techniques can identify tumors less than one-half centimeter in diameter. A combination of regular breast examination by the patient and the physician and periodic mammography offers the best chance of early detection of breast cancer at a time when the tumor is small, axillary lymph nodes are uninvolved, and, consequently, the possibility of curative therapy is high.

Because of normally increased breast density in young women, the detection of very small tumors in this age group may be more difficult. Overall, mammographic interpretation by a qualified radiologist is accurate in about 90% of cases.

INDICATIONS

1. Verification of clinically suspicious lesions before biopsy. (Regardless of mammographic appearance, all palpable breast masses must be biopsied or aspirated).
2. Demonstration of multiple primary lesions or bilateral cancers in a patient who presents with a single palpable mass.
3. Screening of high-risk women: those with a history of previous breast cancer or with breast cancer in the patient's mother, sister, or daughter.
4. General screening of all women over age 50 with an initial baseline examination between age 35 and 40 (Figure 1.6).

PREPARATION

None.

TECHNIQUE

The breast is compressed between the film cassette and a plastic compression device, thus equalizing breast thickness and permitting an even density of the breast to project on film. A low-energy x-ray beam passes through the breast, resulting in the diagnostic image.

At some centers xeromammography is performed. This technique uses x-ray as the energy source but records the image on an electrically charged plate covered with a blue powder. The final image is the result of deposition of the blue powder on paper. There are advantages and disadvantages to both the film and xeromammographic techniques.

RISKS

Questions have been raised regarding the possible oncogenic risk of irradiating asymptomatic women in mammographic screening programs. With current equipment and faster film the radiation dose to the breast parenchyma is only a fraction of what it was just a few years ago. Most authorities consider the oncogenic risk of mammography extremely small if proper guidelines are followed and up-to-date equipment used.

TIME REQUIRED

30–60 minutes.

COST

$

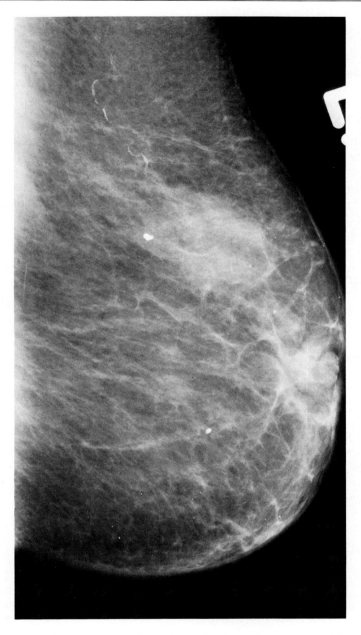

Figure 1.6 *Lateral mammographic view of a breast without evidence of carcinoma. Several benign calcifications are evident. Linear calcifications in the upper portion are vascular in origin, and the dense globular calcifications represent intraductal calcium.*

MYELOGRAPHY

ASSESSMENT

Myelography reliably demonstrates tumors within the spinal canal and spinal cord, both primary and metastatic. If a single disease site is suspected based on clinical findings and plain radiographs, computerized tomography of the spine following water-soluble contrast (metrizamide) injection into the subarachnoid space is ideal. For evaluation of several spinal segments or the entire spinal canal, however, conventional plain film myelography using a nonwater-soluble contrast agent is preferred.

INDICATIONS

1. Evaluation of patients with suspected spinal cord compression or cauda equina syndrome by demonstrating intradural and extradural metastases (Figure 1.7).
2. Evaluation of suspected primary spinal cord tumors (rare).

TECHNIQUE

A lumbar puncture is performed and cerebrospinal fluid obtained for analysis including cytology before contrast is injected through the LP needle into the lumbar subarachnoid space. The patient is tilted into varying positions on a tilt-table, and multiprojectional views are obtained using either conventional x-ray equipment or computerized tomography.

PREPARATION

None.

RISKS

1. Post-LP headache due to cerebrospinal fluid leak.
2. Seizures due to the spill of metrizamide into the calvarium.
3. Arachnoiditis.

28

TIME REQUIRED

1–2 hours.

COST

$$ conventional myelography.
$$$$ myelography with computerized tomography.

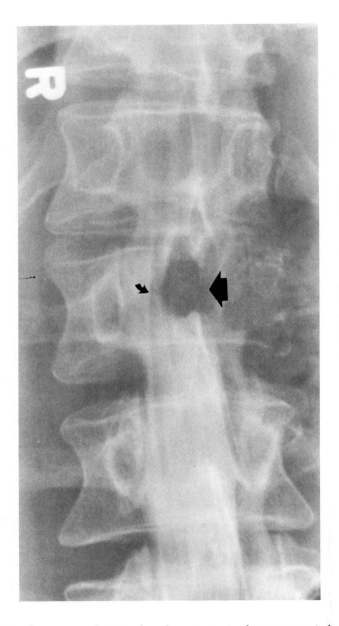

Figure 1.7   *Myelogram with intradural metastasis (large arrow) deviating adjacent nerve root (small arrow).*

NUCLEAR IMAGING: BONE

ASSESSMENT

The radionuclide bone scan provides a much more sensitive method than plain radiography for the early detection of bony metastases. The combination of negative x-ray films with a positive scan is a common finding in patients with early metastatic disease. The isotope scan abnormality may predate plain film findings by as much as 6 months. Serial bone scans are useful in detecting disease progression by showing the appearance of new lesions, but they are not generally useful in following response to therapy. The radiation therapist may obtain helpful information from the bone scan for use in planning treatment for painful bony lesions.

Positive bone scans are seen with various nonmalignant conditions, including arthritis, Paget's disease, fractures, and osteomyelitis, but correlation with the clinical situation and radiographic findings usually prevents confusion. The bone scan may rarely be negative in cases of purely lytic bony lesions, such as those seen in multiple myeloma and occasionally in certain solid tumors. Diffuse uniform involvement of the entire skeleton may rarely be mistaken for a negative study.

INDICATIONS

Detection and assessment of bony metastases (Figure 1.8).

TECHNIQUE

A technetium-99m (^{99m}Tc)-labelled phosphate compound is injected intravenously approximately 2 hours before patient scanning. The phosphate compound avidly seeks sites of active bone metabolism such as those evoked by metastases. Usually the entire body is imaged, although in some centers the distal extremities are omitted. This omission is not recommended, however, since distal extremity metastases, although uncommon, do occur. After viewing the total body scan, the radiologist may request separate filming of suspicious areas of increased photon activity (hot areas). This permits more detailed examination of the abnormal areas and improved anatomic localization.

PREPARATION

None.

RISKS

Allergic reactions have very rarely been encountered.

TIME REQUIRED

3–4 hours.

COST

$$

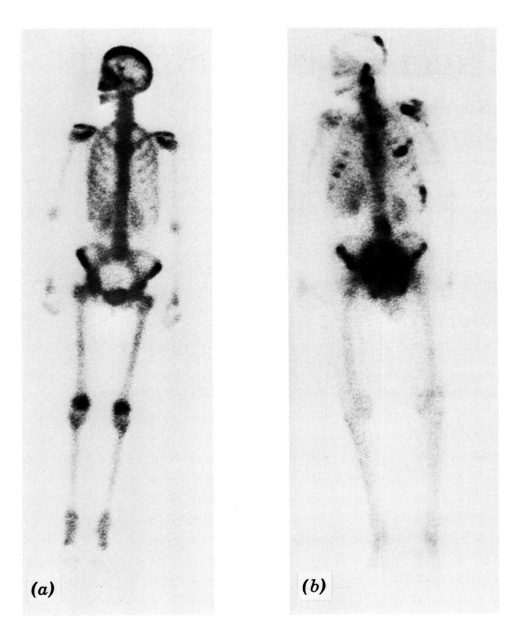

(a)   *(b)*

Figure 1.8 *(a) Normal technetium-99m pyrophosphate bone scan. (b) Bone scan demonstrating multiple areas of increased activity representing metastases in a patient with breast cancer.*

NUCLEAR IMAGING: BRAIN

ASSESSMENT

The sensitivity of the radionuclide brain scan is close to that of computerized tomography for the detection of brain metastases. In most medical centers, however, computerized tomography has almost completely replaced radionuclide scanning for the evaluation of both primary and metastatic lesions. Computerized tomography offers considerably greater anatomic detail and is more useful in the assessment of many benign conditions that may clinically mimic brain tumors.

INDICATIONS

Detection and localization of both primary and metastatic brain tumors.

TECHNIQUE

Technetium-99m DPTA or glucoheptanate is injected intravenously 1 hour before scanning. Multiple gamma camera views of the head, including anterior, posterior, both laterals, and occasionally vertex, are obtained. When posterior fossa lesions are suspected, additional views of that area are taken.

PREPARATION

None.

RISKS

Allergic reactions have very rarely been encountered.

TIME REQUIRED

90–120 minutes.

COST

$$

NUCLEAR IMAGING: GALLIUM

ASSESSMENT

Radionuclide scanning with gallium-67 (^{67}Ga) citrate is used in the staging of lymphomas and bronchogenic carcinomas. The sensitivity of the gallium scan for lung cancer is approximately 90% for disease in the chest but considerably less for distant metastases. In the lymphomas the gallium scan has a sensitivity of 70–80%, higher for the histiocytic lymphomas and lower for the lymphocytic lymphomas.

Following injection, ^{67}Ga is taken up by the liver and axial skeleton and excreted in the colon. It is also taken up by granulocytes, hence its use in detecting inflammatory lesions. Clearly ^{67}Ga is not specific for malignancy, and interpretation of a gallium scan requires knowledge of normal variants, especially bowel accumulation of isotope, and consideration of the possibility of inflammatory processes. Gallium scanning has limited value in the immediate postoperative period because of increased gallium activity at the site of healing.

INDICATIONS

Detection and localization of occult areas of infection (particularly abscesses) and malignancies, especially lymphomas and bronchogenic carcinomas (Figure 1.9).

TECHNIQUE

Gallium-67 citrate is injected intravenously, and scans are obtained 24, 48, and 72 hours later. A scintillation camera records the image, primarily of the thorax and abdomen. If increased activity is seen in the region of the colon, a cleansing enema is given. If the activity persists on serial images, it can then be assumed that the avid site is distinct from bowel and represents a pathologic process. Before gallium scanning a radionuclide liver–spleen scan is performed in order to locate the liver and prevent confusion when evaluating gallium activity in the upper abdomen.

PREPARATION

Bowel preparation is usually not required.

RISKS

Allergic reactions have very rarely been encountered.

TIME REQUIRED

2–3 days. A few minutes on the first day and about 1 hour on each subsequent day.

COST

$$$

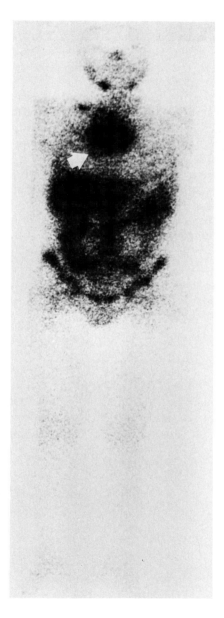

Figure 1.9 Gallium-67 citrate scan with focus of increased activity (arrow) representing mediastinal adenopathy in a patient with lymphoma.

37

NUCLEAR IMAGING: LIVER

ASSESSMENT

In recent years computerized tomography and ultrasonography have all but replaced radionuclide liver scanning in the evaluation of liver metastases. In large part this preference can be explained by the additional information about other abdominal organs (such as pancreas and retroperitoneal lymph nodes) that the newer modalities provide. Nevertheless, liver scanning for the detection of metastases remains a useful tool in certain clinical circumstances.

In the past the liver scan was widely used for routine screening of patients with various extrahepatic malignancies. Fortunately, this habit is waning as physicians recognize the low yield and considerable unreliability of the test in patients without clinical indication of liver involvement.

INDICATIONS

1. Evaluation of the liver for metastases. Not recommended for routine screening in patients with various primary tumors in the absence of specific clinical indications (Figure 1.10).
2. Assessment of spleen size.

TECHNIQUE

Technetium-99m sulfur colloid is injected intravenously about 15 minutes before gamma camera imaging of the upper abdomen. Both the liver and spleen are imaged simultaneously, and multiple projections of both structures are obtained and recorded on film.

PREPARATION

None.

RISKS

Allergic reactions have rarely been encountered.

TIME REQUIRED

30–45 minutes.

COST

$$

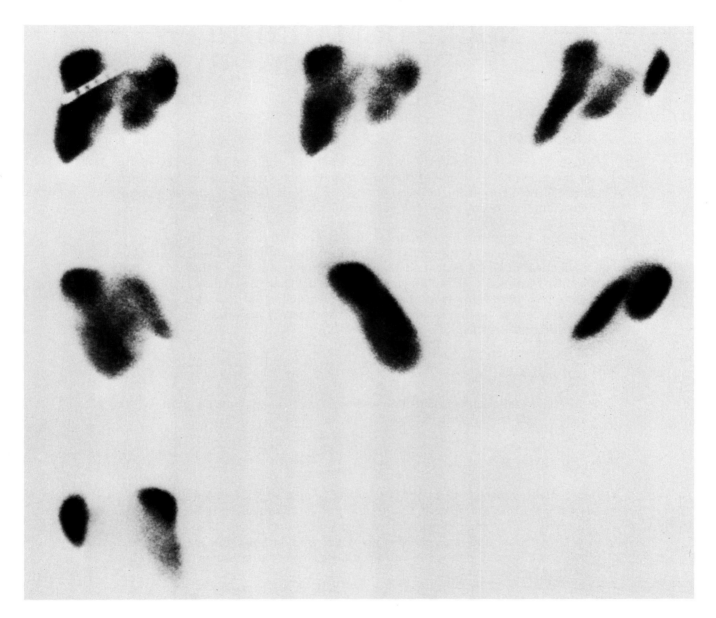

Figure 1.10   Normal multiple view liver scan.

NUCLEAR MAGNETIC RESONANCE SCANNING

ASSESSMENT

Nuclear magnetic resonance (NMR) has been employed in analytical chemistry for the past few decades but has only recently been introduced as a medical imaging tool. The ultimate place of NMR in cancer diagnosis and staging remains unclear at this point, but early results have generated considerable optimism.

Unlike current imaging modalities such as computerized tomography, ultrasonography, and angiography, NMR has the ability to analyze the concentration of specific atomic elements and chemical environments within the body. NMR may also be useful in classifying neoplasms on the basis of metabolic properties. It is hoped that this type of analysis will eventually lead to earlier and more accurate documentation of neoplastic disease than is possible with currently available imaging methods.

INDICATIONS

At present NMR is an experimental method in medical imaging, and indications for its use in cancer patients (and others) have not been defined.

TECHNIQUE

The patient is placed within the core of a large magnet. Radiofrequency signals are directed into the magnetic field, altering the polarization of atoms within the body. The change in polarity of a specific group of atoms in the patient can be detected and presented as an image by computerized manipulation. Reconstruction of the image in various planes, as in computerized tomography, can then be performed.

PREPARATION

None.

RISKS

None currently known.

TIME REQUIRED

1–2 hours.

COST

$$$$ (when available)

PERCUTANEOUS BIOPSY

ASSESSMENT

Once clinical suspicion of malignant disease has been raised, histologic verification must precede therapeutic planning. Until recently, tissue specimens for such verification were obtained by surgical biopsy, exploratory laparotomy, hollow visceral endoscopy (bronchoscopy, gastroscopy, colonoscopy), laparoscopy, mediastinoscopy, and blind percutaneous biopsy of the liver. With the establishment of the "skinny needle" percutaneous biopsy technique by the Japanese and Scandinavians, another tool has become available, often obviating the need for more dangerous invasive methods.

Almost any anatomic site—intrathoracic, intra-abdominal, retroperitoneal—may provide a target for percutaneous biopsy. Tumor masses, solid viscera, and lymph nodes can be readily sampled. Risks are minimal and yields are high, particularly when the biopsy procedure is guided by ultrasonography or computerized tomography.

Because of the possibility of sampling error, the physician can rely only on the results of a positive biopsy. A negative result requires confirmation, usually by surgical biopsy methods.

INDICATION

To provide tissue confirmation of a suspected malignant process in the liver, lung, pleura, pancreas, retroperitoneal lymph nodes, kidney, intra-abdominal masses, and other sites (Figure 1.11).

TECHNIQUE

The target area is first visualized with the appropriate imaging modality: ultrasonography or computerized tomography for a tumor mass or visceral biopsy; fluoroscopy for pleural or pulmonary parenchymal lesions or for previously opacified retroperitoneal lymph nodes.

The skin is prepared with surgical iodine and alcohol and local anesthetic is infiltrated down to pleura or peritoneum. Depending on the site, the biopsy is performed with either aspiration or screw needle technique, the former yielding a cytologic specimen, the latter a tissue or histologic specimen. Two to five samples are obtained and, in many cases, stained and examined by a pathologist immediately so that additional specimens can be obtained at the same sitting if the original material is inadequate.

Although the needle may, and almost certainly does, pass through bowel on the way to many intra-abdominal or retroperitoneal lesions, clinically evident peritonitis does not occur. In fact, percutaneous biopsies may be performed on an outpatient basis, as long as the patient may be observed for several hours following the procedure.

PREPARATION

1. NPO after midnight.
2. Check clotting parameters.
3. Premedicate with 10 mg diazepam and 0.3–0.4 mg atropine IM 30 minutes before the procedure (these agents may be omitted if clinical circumstances—heart disease, glaucoma—warrant).

RISKS

1. Despite the probable penetration of small vascular and alimentary structures, the risk of clinically significant, or even measurable, bleeding or peritoneal contamination is small.
2. Transthoracic biopsy may result in pneumothorax in up to 30% of cases, but therapeutic intervention with tube thoracostomy is necessary only about 10% of the time.

TIME REQUIRED

30–60 minutes. Actual biopsy time is less than 5 minutes; preparation and imaging occupy the balance.

COST

$$

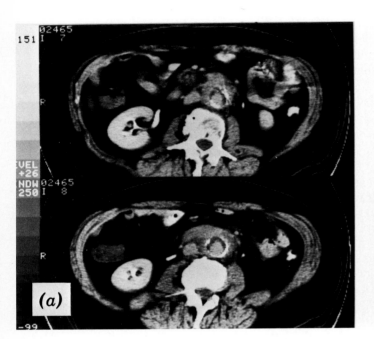
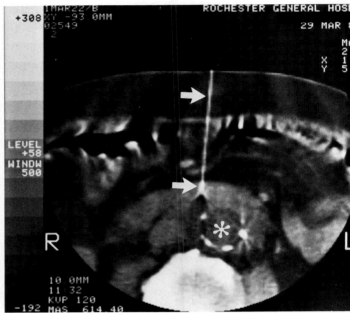

Figure 1.11 (a) Percutaneous biopsy of a para-aortic mass. The needle (arrows) is seen in place just anterior to the aorta (*). Calcifications within the aortic wall define its margins. (b) Percutaneous biopsy of a mass in the head of the pancreas, which proved to be pancreatic carcinoma.

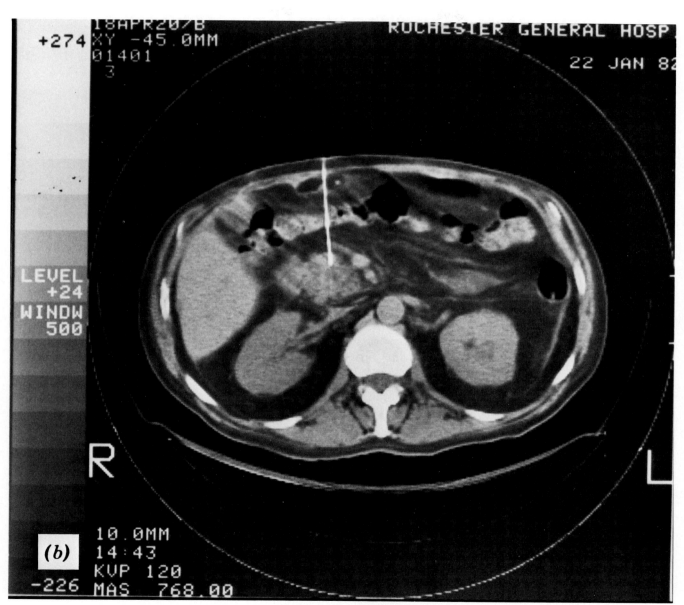

Figure 1.11   (Continued)

PERCUTANEOUS TRANSHEPATIC CHOLANGIOGRAPHY

ASSESSMENT

Percutaneous transhepatic cholangiography (PTC) is the examination of choice for visualizing the biliary system, confirming biliary obstruction, locating the site, and often defining the nature of that obstruction. In a typical case the clinical picture and a noninvasive imaging method (ultrasonography or computerized tomography) lead to a diagnosis of obstructive jaundice and suggest the need for PTC to define the site and predict the probable cause of the obstruction. The percutaneous cholangiogram allows the surgeon to plan preoperatively the best biliary drainage procedure or may precede attempts at percutaneous biliary drainage, as well as percutaneous biopsy of the obstructing lesion.

Percutaneous cholangiography has completely replaced the older large needle cholangiographic technique and has supplanted intravenous cholangiography as well. Endoscopic retrograde cholangiopancreatography (ERCP) is a competing modality for visualization of the biliary system. ERCP requires more time and endoscopic expertise and probably should be reserved for those cases in which ampullary cancer is suspected.

INDICATIONS

1. Verification of biliary obstruction (Figure 1.12).
2. Initial examination before percutaneous biliary drainage.

TECHNIQUE

Under local anesthesia and after appropriate preparation of the skin puncture site, a "skinny" 22-gauge Chiba needle is introduced into a biliary radicle, contrast is injected under fluoroscopic monitoring, and multiprojectional x-ray films of the contrast-filled system are obtained.

If percutaneous biliary drainage is desired, a larger catheter can be inserted into the obstructed system, allowing decompression to take place externally into a collection bag taped to the patient's flank. Alternatively, with the use of a multi-side holed catheter placed with its distal end beyond the site of obstruction, internal biliary drainage may be accomplished.

46

PREPARATION

Broad-spectrum antibiotic coverage before biliary puncture is essential to avoid sepsis. Such coverage should begin 24 hours before the procedure.

RISKS

1. Bacterial sepsis.
2. Bile peritonitis.
3. Hemorrhage.

In most recent series the incidence of serious complications is below 5%. Minor complications, including slight fever, local pain, and relative hypotension, are more common but rarely require treatment.

TIME REQUIRED

1–2 hours.

COST

$$$

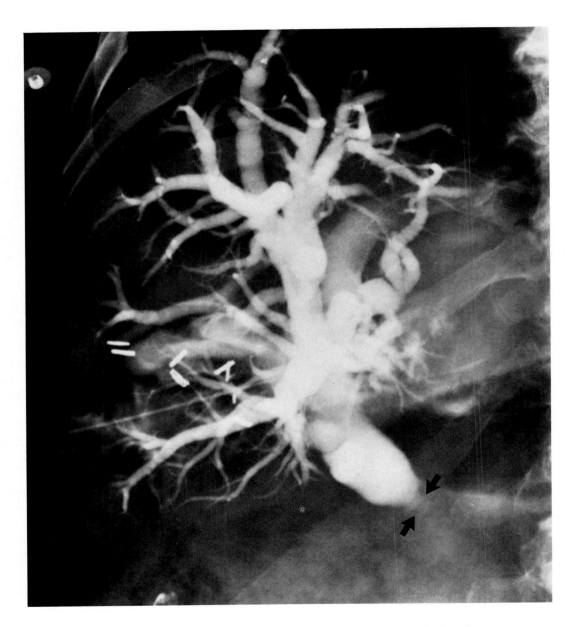

Figure 1.12 *Percutaneous transhepatic cholangiogram with distal common bile duct obstruction (arrows) and proximal dilatation of the biliary system.*

PLAIN FILM TOMOGRAPHY

ASSESSMENT

Plain film tomography has been used for decades as a means of improving a radiographic image by blurring surrounding structures. This method has been employed in the evaluation of pulmonary nodules and mediastinal contours, renal masses, and osseous abnormalities.

Recently, computerized tomography has replaced plain film tomography in many applications. However, plain film tomography may still provide extremely useful information in certain situations at a fraction of the cost of CT.

INDICATIONS

1. Evaluation of specific osseous sites when isotope studies suggest metastatic disease but plain films are confusing due to overlapping structures (Figures 1.13, 1.14).
2. The detection of multiple pulmonary metastases when specific therapy is dependent upon whether single or multiple metastases exist.

TECHNIQUE

Regular radiographs are obtained by keeping the x-ray tube perpendicular to the plane of anatomic interest, while in tomography the tube makes an arc over the area to be studied. This tube motion results in blurring of structures above and beneath the "plane" of interest. Manipulation of the tube motion results in greater or less blurring, and specific motion patterns, such as linear, circular, and hypocycloidal, can be used.

PREPARATION

None.

RISKS

The radiograph is exposed for the duration of the tube motion, and therefore the radiation dose to the patient is greater than with conventional x-rays.

49

TIME REQUIRED

30–60 minutes (depending upon site of examination).

COST

$$

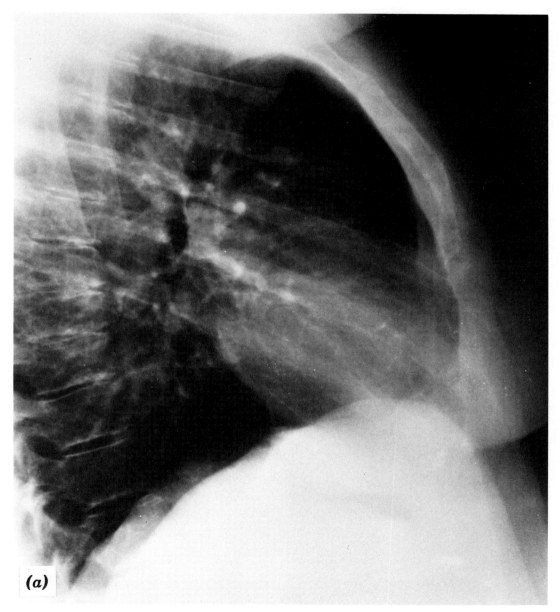

Figure 1.13 (a) Apparently normal lateral view of the chest.

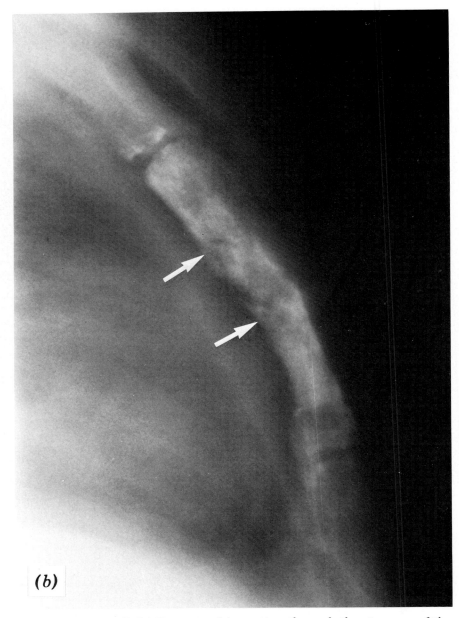

(b)

Figure 1.13 *(Continued) (b) Tomographic section through the sternum of the same patient documenting clinically suspected metastases (arrows).*

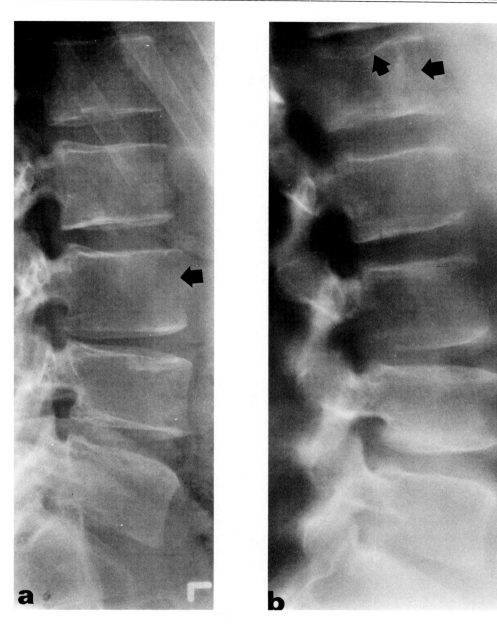

Figure 1.14 (a) Lateral film of the lumbar spine showing destruction of the anterior margin of the third lumbar vertebral body (arrow). (b) Lateral tomogram of the same spine demonstrating unsuspected additional metastatic involvement of the first lumbar vertebral body (arrows).

ULTRASONOGRAPHY

ASSESSMENT

Ultrasonography (or echo) is a rapid, noninvasive, and inexpensive imaging modality. Its chief application in cancer patients is the detection of mass lesions within the peritoneum, pelvis, and retroperitoneum. Liver metastases greater than 1.5 cm in diameter can be demonstrated. Unlike computerized tomography, ultrasonography has the ability to image in a longitudinal plane, as well as in the usual axial or transverse orientation.

In the evaluation of retroperitoneal adenopathy, lymphography and computerized tomography are the preferred imaging procedures. For pelvic masses, however, ultrasonography may be preferable. The ability of ultrasonography to distinguish solid from cystic lesions is often helpful.

INDICATIONS

1. Detection and verification of abdominal, retroperitoneal, and pelvic masses.
2. Demonstration of hepatic metastases (Figures 1.15, 1.16).
3. Guidance for percutaneous biopsy procedures.

TECHNIQUE

A coupling gel, which acts as a conducting medium for the ultrasound waves, is applied to the patient's skin over the area of interest. Ultrasound, a nonionizing form of energy, passes from the crystal at the tip of the transducer through the patient, and the returning echo is collected by the transducer in the detecting mode and then stored on an imaging screen. Permanent film copies can then be made.

PREPARATION

Upper abdomen: Clear liquids for 24 hours before the procedure; then NPO after midnight.
Pelvis: The patient should have a full bladder for optimal imaging and therefore should not void (or should have a Foley catheter clamped) for 4 hours before the study.

RISKS

None.

TIME REQUIRED

30 minutes.

COST

$

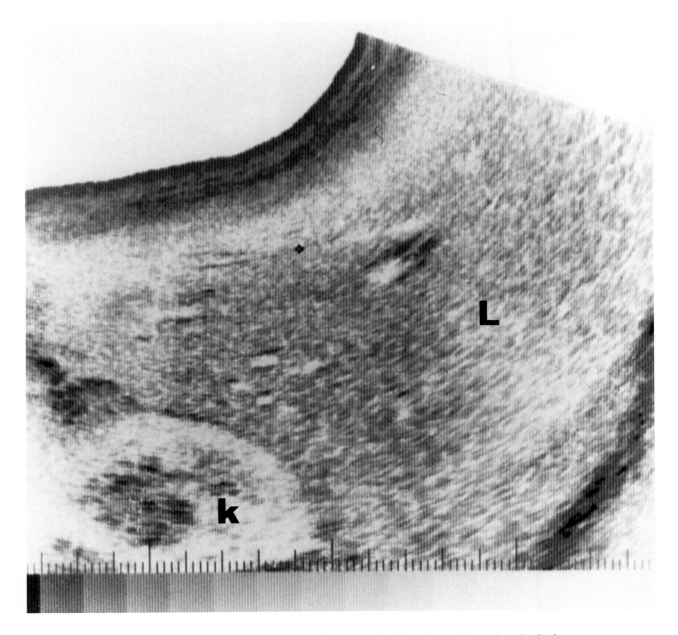

Figure 1.15 *Normal longitudinal ultrasound of the liver (L) and right kidney (k).*

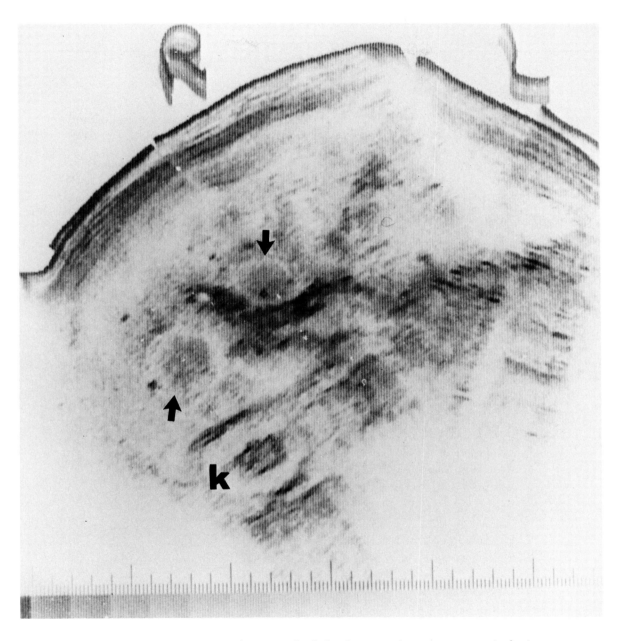

Figure 1.16 *Transverse ultrasound of the liver with two metastatic lesions (arrows).*

UROGRAPHY

ASSESSMENT

Excretory urography is usually the initial examination in cases of suspected renal masses. Additional confirmatory studies, such as ultrasonography, computerized tomography, and angiography, are required.

The urogram no longer has a role in the evaluation of retroperitoneal adenopathy, except in conjunction with the storage (24-hour) phase of a lymphogram.

INDICATIONS

1. First study in the evaluation of hematuria or suspected renal mass.
2. Detection of the presence and level of ureteral obstruction (Figure 1.17).
3. Location of the ureters before major pelvic surgery.

TECHNIQUE

Contrast is injected intravenously and a series of films, including tomograms of the kidneys, is taken to assess excretory function and renal morphology. Subsequent films demonstrate ureteral size and location, and final films evaluate the bladder before and after voiding.

PREPARATION

1. Bowel cleansing as for barium enema.
2. NPO after midnight before the examination.
3. Assure adequate hydration.
4. Assure adequate renal function.

RISKS

1. Iodinated contrast reaction.
2. Renal functional impairment (unlikely in well-hydrated patients).

TIME REQUIRED

60–90 minutes.

COST

$

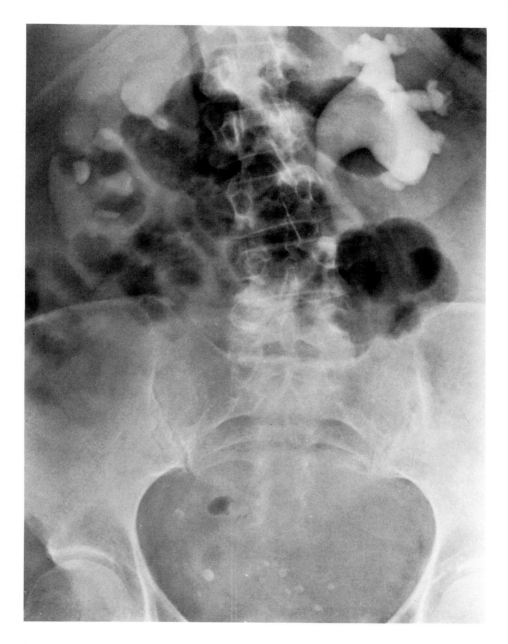

Figure 1.17 Single anterior view from an excretory urogram demonstrating dilated intrarenal collecting systems due to bilateral ureteral obstruction. In this patient the cause was a large ovarian carcinoma.

CHAPTER 2

Radiologic Evaluations by Site

Several regions of the body frequently require assessment for tumor spread, regardless of the primary origin of the tumor. Proper evaluation of these areas demands a knowledge of the strengths and weaknesses of the various imaging modalities that can be brought to bear, as well as an understanding of the usual patterns of spread of each type of cancer.

MEDIASTINAL LYMPH NODES

Mediastinal lymph nodes may be involved by metastatic spread from a variety of primary malignancies, both those arising within the thorax and those with origins elsewhere.

Superior mediastinal and paratracheal lymph nodes are frequently involved with lymphomas. Primary lung cancers, usually following extension to ipsilateral hilar nodes, may spread to ipsilateral or contralateral mediastinal nodes. Breast cancer may spread to the internal mammary lymph node group (Figure 2.1) or to the subcarinal and anterior mediastinal nodes. Other tumors that affect mediastinal nodes with some regularity include carcinomas of the esophagus and testis.

Four major imaging tools are available for evaluation of mediastinal lymph nodes: (1) plain radiography with oblique projections (55°) and barium swallow, (2) plain film tomography, (3) computerized tomography (CT), and (4) gallium scanning.

Bulky mediastinal adenopathy is usually evident on standard posteroanterior (Figure 2.2) and lateral (Figure 2.3) chest films, but 55° oblique views, combined with a barium swallow (Figure 2.4) to mark the esophagus, are more sensitive. Even greater sensitivity (i.e., detection of smaller mediastinal lymph nodes) can be obtained with plain film (Figure 3.64b) or computerized tomography. Computerized tomography can identify lymph nodes 1–2 cm in diameter and is the most sensitive modality for evaluation of the mediastinum (Figure 2.5). However, not every enlarged lymph node harbors tumor; reactive processes, particularly prevalent among lung cancer patients, cannot always be distinguished from metastatic involvement. If such a distinction is critical, mediastinotomy or mediastinoscopy with node biopsies, is essential.

Gallium scanning can be used to detect occult mediastinal involvement with lung cancer or lymphoma (Figure 1.9). The specificity of this modality is low, however, and false-positive results can be seen with inflammatory diseases, sarcoid, and other nonmalignant conditions.

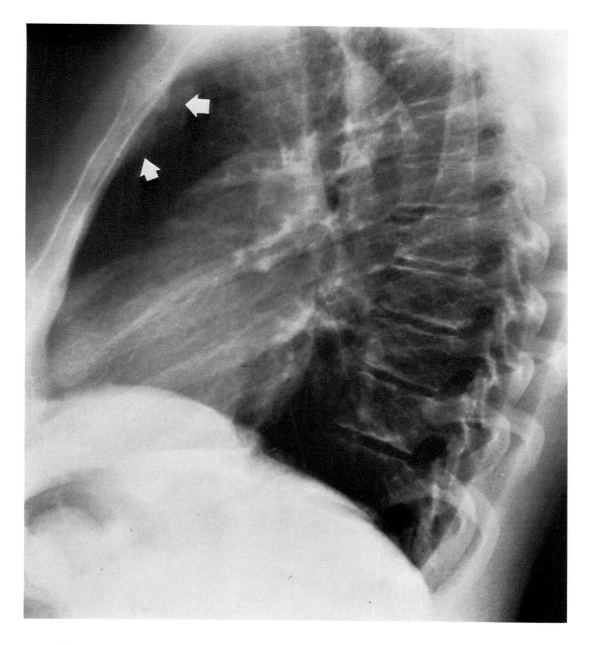

Figure 2.1 *Lateral chest film with subtle internal mammary lymphadenopathy (arrows) in a woman with breast cancer.*

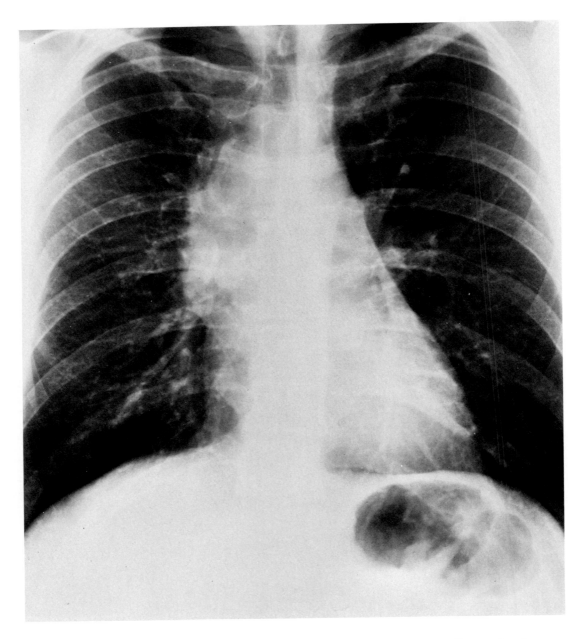

Figure 2.2 *Posteroanterior chest film demonstrating right mediastinal adenopathy in a patient with Hodgkin's disease.*

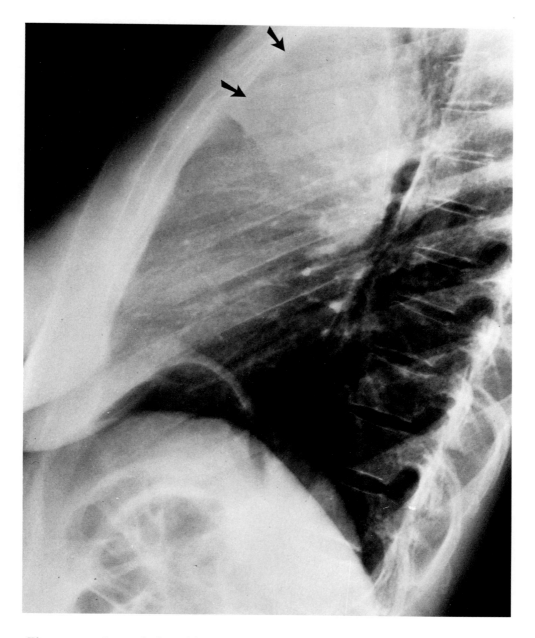

Figure 2.3 *Lateral chest film with an anterior mediastinal mass (arrows) consisting of lymph nodes involved with Hodgkin's disease.*

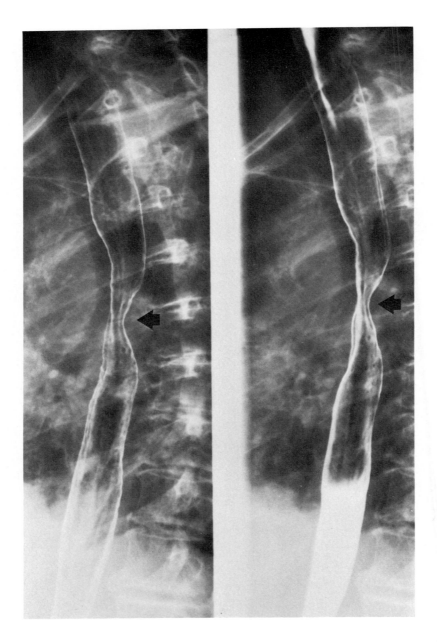

Figure 2.4 Portion of a lateral chest film with barium swallow showing subtle indentation of the esophagus (arrow), presumably due to adenopathy in a woman with breast cancer.

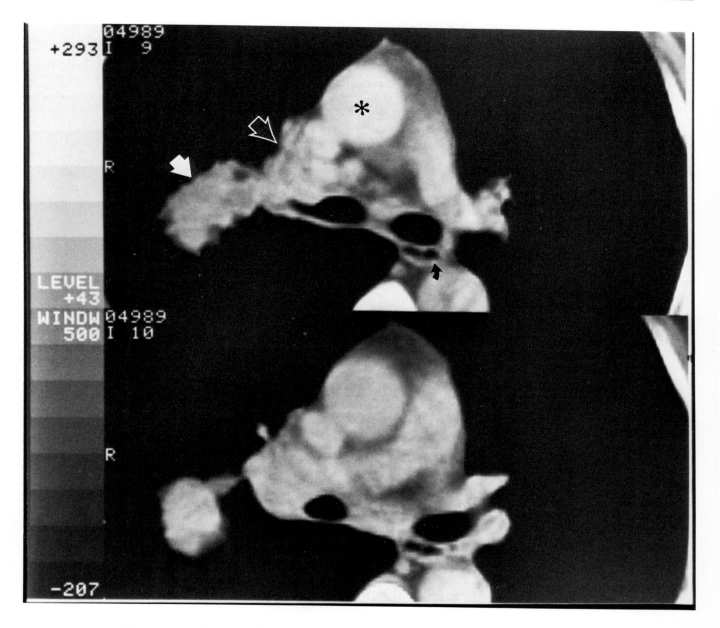

Figure 2.5 *Magnified view of the upper thorax with computerized tomography. Mediastinal adenopathy (open arrow) is seen adjacent to a primary lung cancer (white arrow). The ascending aorta (*) and esophagus (curved arrow) are marked for identification.*

67

PULMONARY NODULES

The lungs are among the most common sites of distant metastasis, and pulmonary evaluation is almost an invariable requirement in the work-up of the patient with newly diagnosed malignant disease. The detection of pulmonary metastases alters the management of the cancer patient, particularly if therapy with curative intent had been anticipated.

Imaging modalities employed in assessing the lungs for metastases include multiprojectional plain x-ray films, plain film whole lung tomography, and computerized tomography. These techniques must respond to two questions in every cancer patient: Are pulmonary nodules present, and, if present, do they represent tumor (primary or secondary) or another etiology?

Plain films often suffice to determine whether metastases are present; with a high quality posteroanterior and lateral examination, metastases can be reliably excluded. Whole lung plain film tomography and computerized tomography offer a small increment in sensitivity above that of plain films. In some circumstances this added sensitivity is important. Certain tumors metastasize early and commonly to the lungs—sarcomas, melanomas, germ cell testicular carcinomas—and appropriate therapy depends on full and accurate assessment, making whole lung tomography by plain film or CT a significant part of the evaluation of these patients. On the other hand, such careful assessment is unwarranted if therapy will proceed regardless of whether asymptomatic pulmonary metastases are detected. For example, an obstructing colon cancer requires palliative surgery whether or not pulmonary metastasis has occurred, and carcinoma of breast metastatic to bone and liver requires systemic chemotherapy whether or not occult pulmonary nodules are present. Under these and similar circumstances the added sensitivity obtainable with lung tomography is irrelevant to the care of the patient.

Lung tomography by plain film or CT technique is also valuable in evaluating individual pulmonary nodules for the specific characteristics of malignancy or benignity. The presence of central calcification is a sign of a benign lung mass, and the density of a lesion as measured by CT imparts an indication of its benign or malignant nature. In addition, the mediastinum can be assessed, if indicated, at the time of the pulmonary study.

Histologic confirmation of the presence of pulmonary metastases is often required and may be accomplished by percutaneous biopsy under radiologic guidance, transbronchial biopsy, or thoracotomy. Such confirmation may be necessary to distinguish a benign from a malignant nodule and to exclude the possibility of synchronous primary tumors (two independent cancers occurring in the same patient at the same time). A solitary pulmonary nodule in a patient with an extrapulmonary malignancy may not necessarily represent a metastasis but rather a primary lung cancer.

HEPATIC MASSES

Tumors from almost any site of origin may metastasize to the liver. Identification of liver metastases, in a patient thought to have localized disease, makes radical treatment of the primary tumor with curative intent inappropriate. For example, nephrectomy for renal cell carcinoma or amputation for osteogenic sarcoma would both be unjustified if liver metastases were documented. On the other hand, an obstructing carcinoma of the sigmoid colon requires palliative surgery whether or not liver metastases are present, and an unresectable carcinoma of the lung causing cough, hemoptysis, and chest pain under most circumstances should receive palliative irradiation whether or not hepatic metastases have occurred. Clearly the importance of determining whether liver metastases are present varies greatly with the clinical situation.

Three imaging modalities are available for hepatic assessment: radionuclide liver scanning, ultrasonography, and computerized tomography. The size threshold for reliable detection of hepatic masses is approximately 2 cm and is about the same for all three techniques. Smaller lesions can be identified with ultrasonography and computerized tomography, but, unless accompanied by larger lesions or multiple additional masses, a definite diagnosis of liver metastasis cannot be made on the basis of one or a few tiny hepatic nodules.

The isotope liver scan is most reliable when focal defects within the liver parenchyma are identified (Figure 3.22). The larger each individual lesion and the greater their number, the greater the degree of assurance in diagnosing hepatic involvement. Diffuse infiltration of the liver by tumor, producing a pattern of inhomogeneous uptake on scan, is difficult to distinguish from non-malignant hepatic parenchymal disease.

Computerized tomography (Figure 2.6), with or without enhancing contrast injection, reliably detects metastatic liver disease. Because computerized tomography is frequently performed for staging of intra-abdominal primary tumors, hepatic assessment during the same examination is highly cost-effective. Computerized tomography performed solely to detect liver metastases, however, is rather expensive, particularly in comparison with the lower cost of ultrasonography and radionuclide scanning.

Both isotope and computerized tomographic scanning may yield false-positive results, especially when cystic disease of the liver is present. Ultrasonography may be helpful in distinguishing benign cysts from metastatic nodules.

If the finding of metastatic involvement of the liver will significantly alter therapy, histologic confirmation may be indicated. In the past this was accomplished with closed needle biopsy, peritoneoscopy with directed liver biopsies, or laparotomy. In recent years, however, needle aspiration cytology under ultrasound or computerized tomographic guidance has become the simplest, most direct method for obtaining a tissue diagnosis.

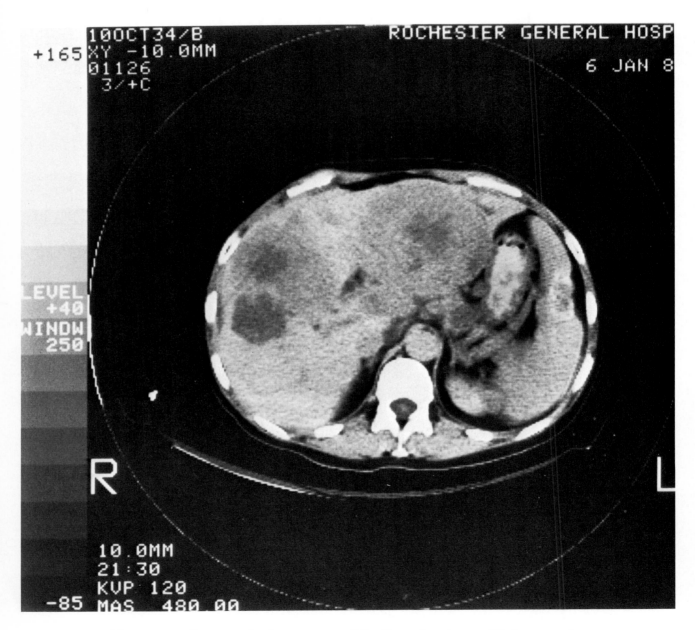

Figure 2.6 Computerized tomogram of the liver showing multiple parenchymal metastases.

OBSTRUCTIVE JAUNDICE

Juandice is a relatively frequent presenting complaint among cancer patients and may arise as a consequence of hepatic replacement with metastatic tumor or of extrahepatic biliary obstruction due to carcinoma of the pancreas, duodenum, ampulla of Vater, or bile ducts. Involvement of porta hepatis lymph nodes with metastatic tumor (breast cancer, lymphomas, gastrointestinal cancer, and others) occasionally produces obstructive jaundice as well.

Evaluation of the jaundiced patient requires a distinction between hepatic metastases and extrahepatic obstruction. Either ultrasonography or computerized tomography can detect parenchymal metastases or distended biliary radicles (Figures 3.41, 3.42), the hallmark of extrahepatic obstruction. Both modalities also allow examination of the head of the pancreas for possible primary carcinoma arising there (Figures 3.24, 3.25). If a pancreatic mass or hepatic nodules are identified, percutaneous biopsy under CT (Figure 1.11b) or ultrasound guidance should follow. If extrahepatic biliary obstruction without apparent pancreatic mass is documented, percutaneous transhepatic cholangiography (PTC) (Figure 3.27) or endoscopic retrograde cholangiopancreatography (ERCP) (Figure 3.26) should follow; these techniques will locate the exact site of biliary obstruction and in some cases indicate the probable cause. The choice between ERCP and PTC depends upon physician preference, endoscopic expertise, and patient tolerance. Either examination can be used to guide percutaneous needle biopsy of any mass visualized.

Technetium-99m HIDA scanning of the biliary system has recently been introduced into medical imaging. Its primary role is in the diagnosis of acute cholecystitis, but it may detect common bile duct obstruction as well. Partial obstruction may go undetected by this examination, however, and it yields no information regarding the cause of the obstruction.

Recently, interventional radiologic techniques have been developed that allow percutaneous drainage of a biliary system obstructed due to cancer. Drainage can be directed externally to a collection bag taped to the patient's skin or internally through an indwelling bypass catheter or stent. Such percutaneous drainage procedures may obviate the need for surgical intervention in a patient with a limited life expectancy.

RETROPERITONEAL AND PELVIC LYMPH NODES

A wide variety of cancers may involve the retroperitoneal and pelvic lymph nodes, making assessment of these regions one of the most common problems in oncologic diagnosis and staging. Solid tumors arising in the pelvis—carcinomas of the rectum, bladder, prostate, cervix, and endometrium—tend to spread to the lymph nodes in the pelvis and para-aortic regions in a sequential, predictable fashion. Primary gastrointestinal cancers—carcinomas of the pancreas, stomach, and esophagus—characteristically spread to the celiac and upper para-aortic nodes. Lymphomas may involve the retroperitoneal and pelvic nodes in one or several areas and typically cause massive nodal replacement and consequent bulky adenopathy. Solid tumors, on the other hand, usually cause only partial replacement as tumor emboli grow within the marginal sinuses of the node, and therefore do not regularly produce massive enlargement of involved nodes (testicular carcinomas are an exception).

These lymph node areas can be imaged with lymphography, computerized tomography, and ultrasonography. Both computerized tomography (Figure 2.7) and ultrasonography (Figure 2.8) detect enlarged lymph nodes and require a 1–2 cm size threshold for visualization. Lymphography, on the other hand, enables lymph nodes of normal size to be visualized and can identify abnormalities of lymph node architecture within nodes of normal or increased size.

For these reasons, lymphography is often more sensitive than ultrasonography or computerized tomography for identification of lymph node involvement with solid tumors. However, visualization of the upper para-aortic lymph nodes with lymphography is uncertain, since insufficient amounts of contrast may reach this area. Therefore examination of the upper para-aortic region is more reliably accomplished with ultrasonography or computerized tomography.

Computerized tomography is the modality of choice for assessing bulky retroperitoneal adenopathy (lymphomas, testicular carcinomas) and high para-aortic, retrocrural, and retrocaval lymph node areas. Ultrasonography is not sufficiently reliable for routine use in lymph node staging, but may be helpful in assessing the upper para-aortic nodes and bulky adenopathy in other areas. The low relative cost of ultrasonography makes this modality a good choice for serial evaluations of an abnormal node or nodes in response to therapy.

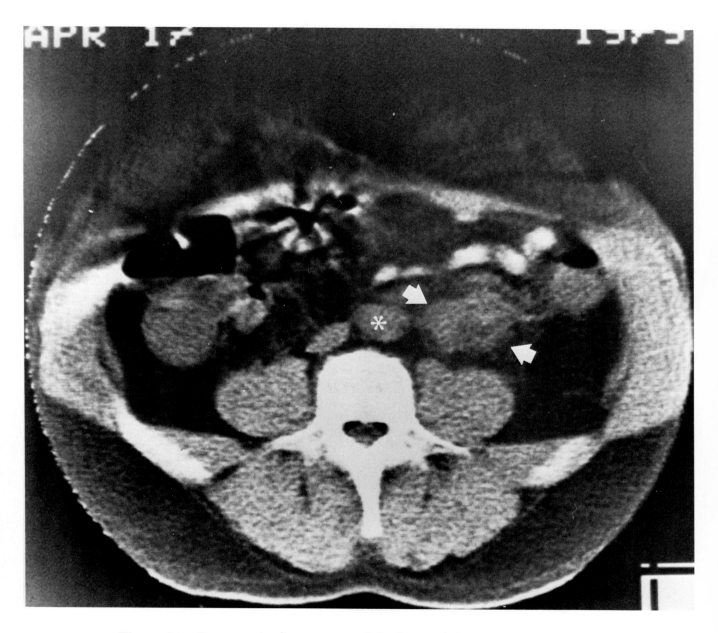

Figure 2.7 Computerized tomogram of the lower abdomen with lymphadenopathy (arrows) adjacent to the aorta (*).

73

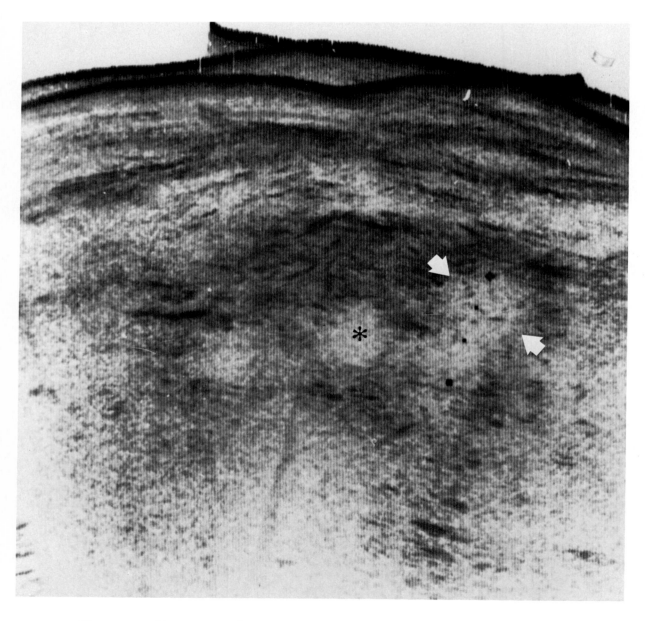

Figure 2.8 Transverse ultrasound of the same location also demonstrating adenopathy (arrows) lateral to the aorta (*).

PELVIC MASSES

Many primary cancers arise within the pelvis. In men carcinomas of the prostate, rectum, and bladder predominate, while in women ovarian, endometrial, and cervical cancers occur in addition to bladder and rectal carcinomas. Metastatic disease from primary tumors of the gastrointestinal tract (and occasionally from breast cancer, lymphomas, and other tumors) may involve the pelvis by the so-called "drop" route where malignant cells are deposited within the peritoneal cavity and settle in the most dependent location, often the pouch of Douglas in women.

The pelvic organs and contents may be studied by several methods including physical examination (often under anesthesia), barium examination of the small and large bowel, ultrasonography, computerized tomography, and direct vision with laparoscopy, cystoscopy, and protosigmoidoscopy.

Barium study is an excellent tool when intraluminal or mucosal lesions are anticipated, such as in patients with rectal bleeding or bowel obstruction. In the staging evaluation of genitourinary cancers, however, barium study can only indicate displacement of bowel due to mass effect and offers no information on the origin or extent of the mass. For these tumors ultrasonography or computerized tomography are particularly useful.

Ultrasonography can often determine the site of origin of a pelvic mass (Figure 3.68) and detect the presence of ascites, hydronephrosis, and bulky adenopathy. The liver can be assessed at the same time, although liver metastasis from an early stage gynecologic tumor would be unusual.

Compared with ultrasonography, computerized tomography offers greater resolution in the detection of local spread of pelvic tumors (Figure 3.69) and pelvic lymph node involvement (Figure 3.71). Ascites, hydronephrosis, retroperitoneal adenopathy, and liver metastases can also be evaluated during the same examination.

Direct visualization of the intraperitoneal pelvic structures can be accomplished with laparoscopy, and biopsies can be performed of visualized lesions. Ascites, extensive adhesions, and mesenteric tumor bulk may interfere with the procedure. Laparoscopy is of particular utility in the evaluation of suspected ovarian cancer.

CHAPTER 3

Diagnosis and Staging of Primary Malignancies

LUNG CANCER

INCIDENCE

135,000 projected new cases in the U.S. in 1983
117,000 deaths
16% of new cancers in Americans
Male:female ratio 2.29

Lung cancer accounts for over 25% of all cancer deaths in the United States and is by far the most common cause of cancer deaths in American males (Figure 3.1).

EPIDEMIOLOGY

Cigarette smoking is the main epidemiologic factor contributing to the etiology of lung cancer. Smokers have 20–30 times greater risk of developing lung cancer than nonsmokers. Occupational exposure to certain particulate metals, radiation, and air pollution are also associated with an increased risk of lung cancer.

PATHOLOGY (Figure 3.2)

Lung cancer is classified into four major pathologic types.

Epidermoid Carcinoma

35–40% of all lung cancers
Central location
Frequently causes obstruction, atelectasis, pneumonia
Most common type to cavitate
Highest resectability rate
Metastasizes late

Adenocarcinoma

20–30% of all lung cancers
Small peripheral tumor
May arise in previous scar or granuloma
Metastasizes relatively early

Small Cell Undifferentiated Carcinoma

15–25% of all lung cancers
Frequent hilar and mediastinal adenopathy at the time of diagnosis
Rarely resectable for cure
Early hematogenous and lymphatic spread

Large Cell Undifferentiated Carcinoma

10–15% of all lung cancers
Large peripheral tumor
Intermediate propensity for metastasis

TUMOR COMPARTMENT

Tumor Signs and Symptoms

Cough	Rib pain
Hemoptysis	Dyspnea
Chest pain	Recurrent laryngeal nerve paralysis
Atelectasis	Horner's syndrome
Pneumonia	Brachial plexus syndrome

Tissue Diagnosis

Percutaneous transthoracic needle aspirate and biopsy for a peripheral lesion
Sputum cytology; bronchoscopy with brushing, washings, and biopsy for a central lesion
Thoracentesis with pleural fluid cytology and/or closed pleural biopsy if pleural effusion present
Thoracotomy may be necessary in those cases in which less invasive techniques fail

Tumor Staging

Plain film or computerized tomography of nearby pleura (Figure 3.3) or mediastinum (may upgrade a lesion from T1 to T2 or T3)
Rib films for lesions that extend to pleura (may upgrade a T2 lesion to T3)
Bronchoscopy, in patients with central lesions, defines tumor distance from carina (T2 versus T3)

79

LYMPH NODE COMPARTMENT

Lymph Node Signs and Symptoms

Superior vena cava syndrome

Dysphagia due to esophageal compression

Recurrent laryngeal nerve paralysis

Pleural effusion due to obstruction of mediastinal lymphatics

Phrenic nerve paralysis

Tissue Diagnosis

Scalene node biopsy is only necessary when a tissue diagnosis cannot be made on the primary tumor. It is particularly useful when the node is palpable.

Mediastinoscopy/mediastinotomy is useful when a tissue diagnosis cannot be made on the primary tumor *and* mediastinal adenopathy is suspected (Figure 3.4).

Lymph Node Staging

Barium esophagram can be used in patients with dysphagia to demonstrate extrinsic compression of the esophagus by enlarged mediastinal nodes.

Plain film or computerized tomography of the mediastinum may upgrade to N2. However, this finding in a patient who is otherwise a candidate for curative surgery should be confirmed with mediastinoscopy or mediastinotomy, since falsely positive imaging of mediastinal nodes can occur.

Gallium scanning may demonstrate mediastinal node involvement.

Mediastinoscopy/mediastinotomy can detect occult mediastinal lymph node metastasis, thus yielding critical information on the feasibility of surgical resection for cure.

METASTASIS COMPARTMENT

Early Stage

In patients who present with stage I or II (potentially resectable) non-small cell lung cancer, the evaluation for metastatic disease should be guided by patient symptoms. In the asymptomatic patient, extensive imaging is unwarranted. On the other hand, patient symptoms and physical findings suggestive of metastatic disease require evaluation with the appropriate diagnostic studies. For example, a patient complaining of headaches should undergo a CT scan of the brain, and a patient with tender hepatomegaly must have liver function tests and hepatic imaging before surgery (Figure 3.5).

Patients with small cell carcinoma, regardless of stage, are presumed to have metastatic disease and are not candidates for curative resections.

Advanced Stage

Distant metastasis in patients with lung cancer, either at the time of initial presentation or later in the course of the disease, typically involves liver, bone, lung, distant lymph nodes, pericardium, brain, skin, bone marrow, and numerous other sites.

TNM CLASSIFICATION OF LUNG CANCER

T: Primary Tumor (Figure 3.6)

TX   Tumor proven by the presence of malignant cells in bronchopulmonary secretions but not visualized roentgenographically or bronchoscopically, or any tumor that cannot be assessed

T0   No evidence of primary tumor

TIS   Carcinoma in situ

T1   Tumor 3.0 cm or less in greatest diameter, surrounded by lung or visceral pleura, and without evidence of invasion proximal to a lobar bronchus at bronchoscopy

T2   Tumor more than 3.0 cm in greatest diameter, or a tumor of any size that either invades the visceral pleura or has associated atelectasis or obstructive pneumonitis extending to the hilar region. At bronchoscopy, the proximal extent of demonstrable tumor must be within a lobar bronchus or at least 2.0 cm distal to the carina. Any associated atelectasis or obstructive pneumonitis must involve less than an entire lung and there must be no pleural effusion.

T3   Tumor of any size with direct extension into an adjacent structure such as the parietal pleura or the chest wall, the diaphragm, or the mediastinum and its contents; or a tumor demonstrable bronchoscopically to involve a main bronchus less than 2.0 cm distal to the carina; or any tumor with atelectasis or obstructive pneumonitis of an entire lung or pleural effusion (whether or not malignant cells are found).

N: Regional Lymph Nodes (Figure 3.7)

N0   No demonstrable metastasis to regional lymph nodes

N1   Metastasis to lymph nodes in the peribronchial or the ipsilateral hilar region, or both, including direct extension

N2   Metastasis to lymph nodes in the mediastinum

M: Distant Metastasis (Figure 3.8)

MX   Not assessed

M0   No known distant metastasis

M1   Distant metastasis present

TNM STAGING OF LUNG CANCER

Occult Carcinoma TX N0 M0	Occult carcinoma with bronchopulmonary secretions containing malignant cells but without other evidence of the primary tumor or evidence of metastasis to the regional lymph nodes or distant metastasis
Stage I: TIS N0 M0	 Carcinoma in situ
T1 N0 M0 T1 N1 M0 T2 N0 M0	Tumor that can be classified T1 without any metastasis or with metastasis to the lymph nodes in the peribronchial or ipsilateral hilar region only, or a tumor that can be classified T2 without any metastasis to nodes or distant metastasis
Stage II: T2 N1 M0	Tumor classified as T2 with metastasis to the lymph nodes in the peribronchial or ipsilateral hilar region only
Stage III: T3 with any N or M N2 with any T or M M1 with any T or N	Any tumor more extensive than T2, or any tumor with metastasis to the lymph nodes in the mediastinum, or any tumor with distant metastasis

CRITERIA FOR INOPERABILITY OF LUNG CANCER
(Figure 3.9)

1. Small cell histology
2. Any distant metastasis (M1)

3. Any mediastinal adenopathy (N2)

   In addition, contralateral hilar adenopathy, superior vena cava obstruction, phrenic nerve paralysis, or recurrent laryngeal nerve paralysis

4. Any T3 lesion

   Extension to chest wall, parietal pleura, diaphragm, mediastinum

   Tumor within 2 cm of the carina

   Tumor associated with atelectasis or obstructive pneumonitis of an entire lung or pleural effusion

   Note: In some medical centers not all T3 lesions are considered inoperable.

PATIENT EVALUATION DIAGRAM

See Figure 3.10.

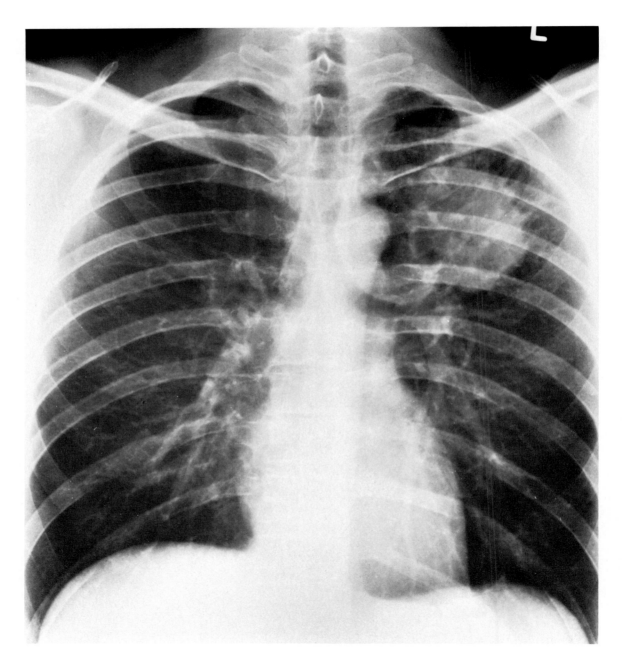

Figure 3.1 *Large cell anaplastic carcinoma of the left upper lobe.*

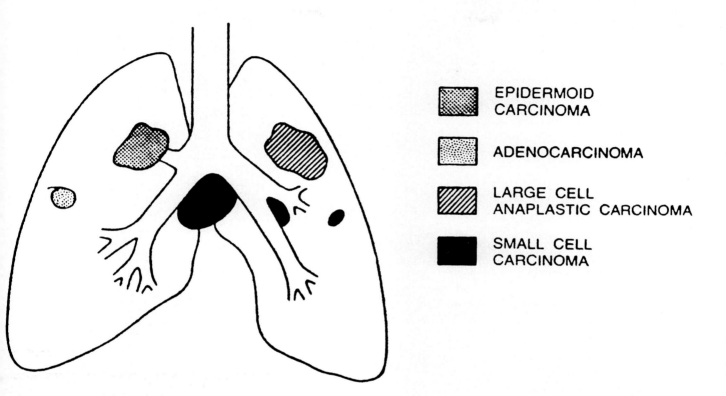

Figure 3.2 *Typical radiographic presentation of the major histologic types of lung cancer.*

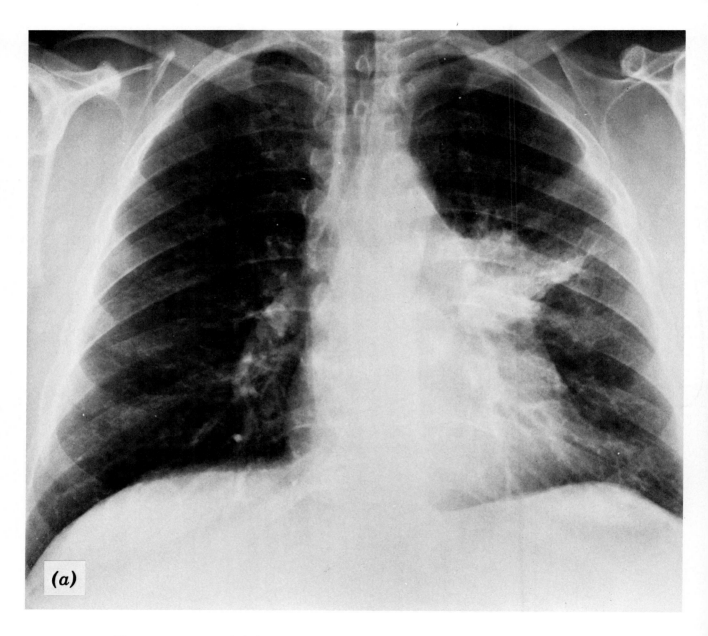

Figure 3.3 (a) Left hilar carcinoma with irregular lateral margin. (b) Plain film tomogram of the left hilar tumor (*) and tumor extension (arrows) to nearby pleura (T3 lesion).

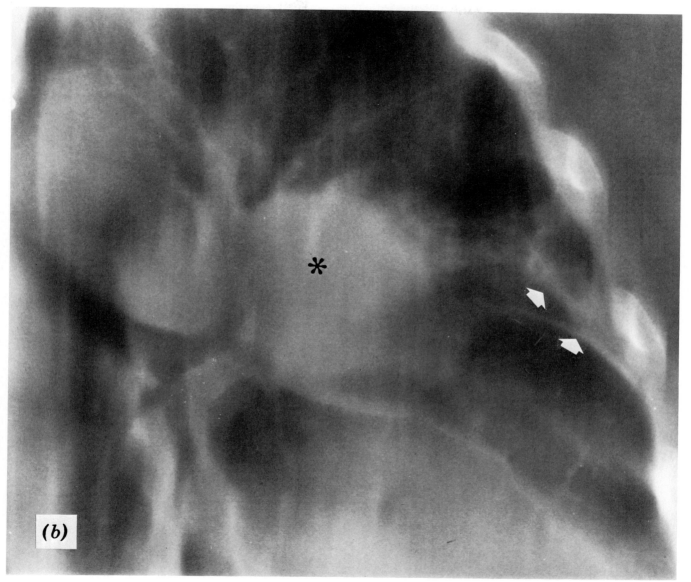

Figure 3.3 (Continued)

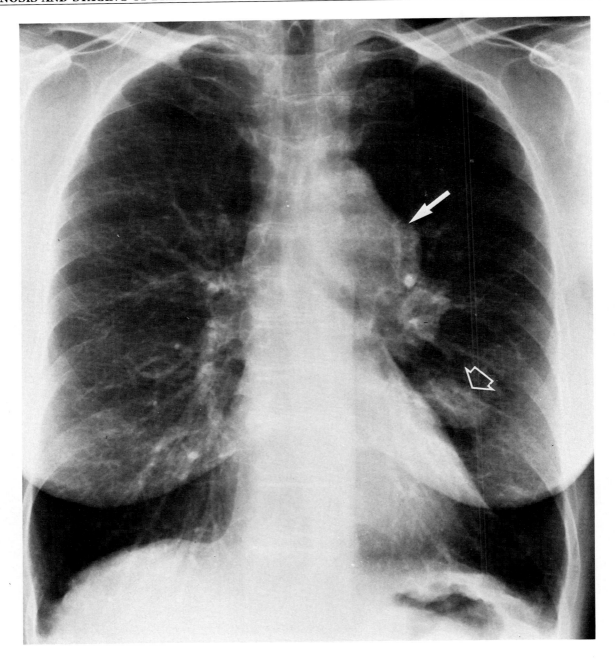

Figure 3.4 *Small cell carcinoma in the left lower lobe (open arrow) with associated mediastinal adenopathy (solid arrow).*

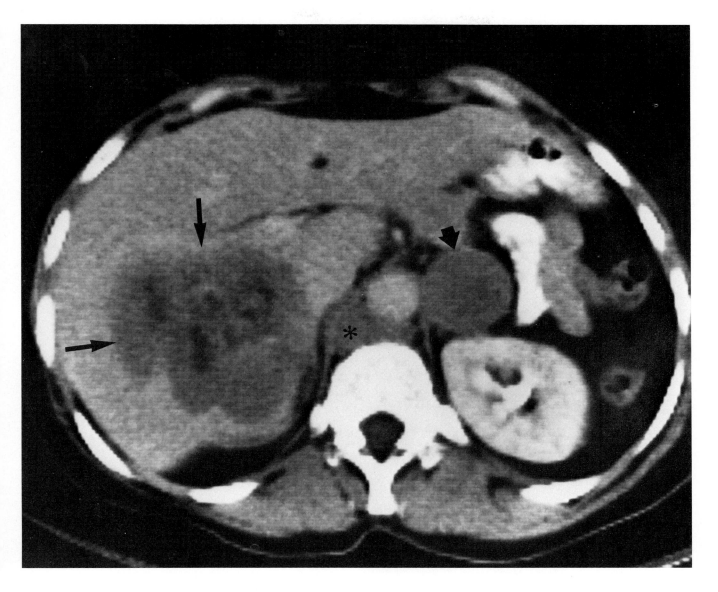

Figure 3.5 *Computerized tomogram of the upper abdomen documenting clinically suspected liver metastasis (long arrows), as well as retrocrural lymphadenopathy (*) and left adrenal metastasis (short arrow).*

89

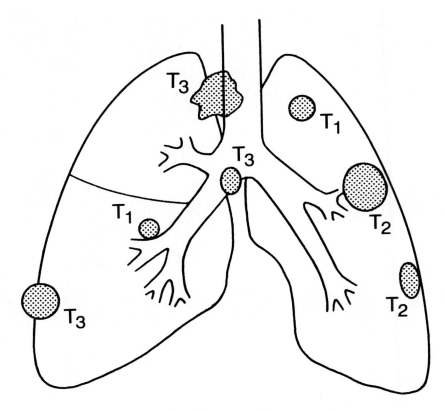

Figure 3.6 Tumor (T) classification of lung cancer.

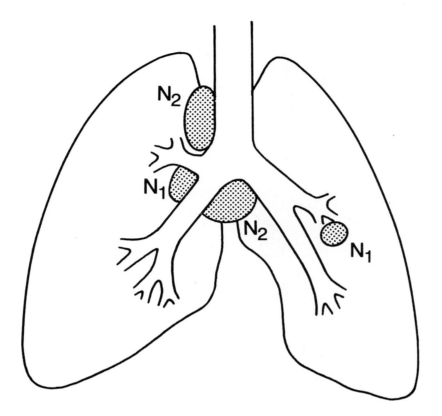

Figure 3.7 Lymph node (N) classifiction of lung cancer.

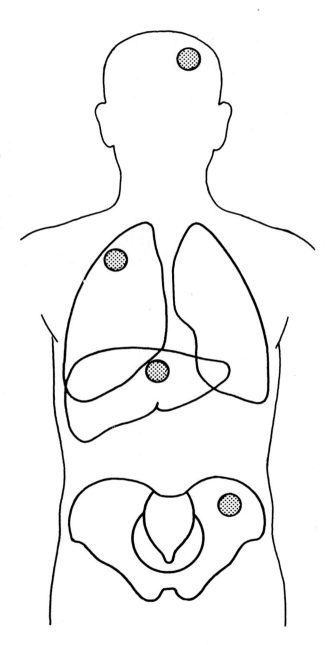

Figure 3.8 Distant metastasis (M) classification of lung cancer.

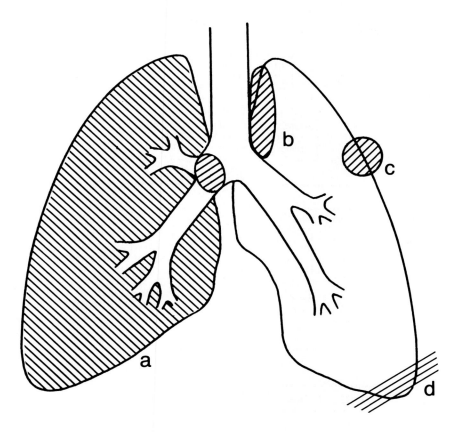

Figure 3.9 *Radiographic manifestations of inoperable lung cancer. a, atelec-tasis; b, mediastinal adenopathy; c, transpleural tumor extension; d, malignant pleural effusion.*

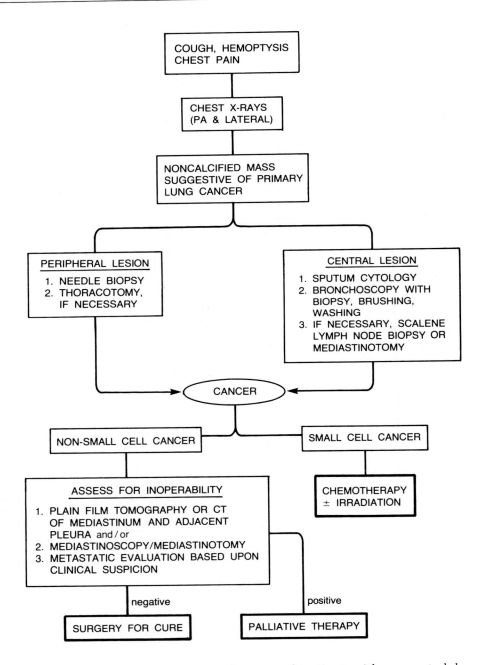

Figure 3.10 *Flow diagram for evaluation of patient with suspected lung cancer.*

BREAST CANCER

INCIDENCE

114,900 projected new cases in the U.S. in 1983

37,500 deaths

13% of new cancers in Americans

Female:male ratio 124:1

Most common cause of cancer deaths in American women

Approximately 1 in every 14 women in the U.S. will develop breast cancer (Figure 3.11)

EPIDEMIOLOGY

Low Risk: Early pregnancy (<18)

                 Multiple pregnancies

                 Castration at an early age

                 Japanese and other Asian women

High Risk: Breast cancer in a close female relative

                 Exposure to ionizing radiation

                 Early menarche and late menopause

                 American women

PATHOLOGY

Infiltrating duct carcinoma (Figure 3.12): 70–80%

Infiltrating lobular carcinoma (often multicentric, sometimes bilateral): 8–10%

Medullary carcinoma: 4–5%

Other and mixed varieties: 7–12%

Inflammatory carcinoma: 1–2%

TUMOR COMPARTMENT

Tumor Signs and Symptoms

Painless mass

Bloody nipple discharge

Swollen, tender, erthematous breast (inflammatory carcinoma)
Ulcerated mass
Asymptomatic, detected by mammographic screening

Tissue Diagnosis

Incisional or excisional biopsy (tissue to be submitted for estrogen receptor analysis as well as pathology)
Needle aspiration cytology (Figure 3.13)

Tumor Staging

Physical examination: tumor size, fixation, skin involvement or edema, inflammatory carcinoma
Mammography: performed to detect other lesions in addition to the clinically evident lesion

LYMPH NODE COMPARTMENT

Lymph Node Signs and Symptoms

Palpable axillary adenopathy
Palpable supra- or infraclavicular adenopathy

Lymph Node Staging

Physical examination of axillary nodes has a high false-positive and false-negative rate
Surgical axillary staging

METASTASIS COMPARTMENT

Early Stage

In patients who present with stage I or stage II breast cancer the incidence of occult metastatic disease is very low. In the absence of clinical indications, routine screening with liver, bone, and brain scans or other procedures is not recommended. However, some oncologists do suggest a bone scan for use as a baseline for comparison with future examinations, particularly in patients with stage II disease. A bone scan with a solitary abnormality (Figure 3.14a) in an asymptomatic patient with early stage breast cancer cannot be accepted as proof of metastasis unless confirmed by x-ray film (Figure 3.14b) or biopsy.

Advanced Stage

Distant metastases in a patient with breast cancer typically involve lymph nodes (Figure 3.15), skin, bone (Figure 3.16), pleura, liver, lung, bone marrow, and brain. Unusual sites of metastasis include gastric mucosa, porta hepatis lymph node causing obstructive jaundice, scalp, and ureter, among others. It is not unusual for a patient with an advanced local lesion (T3 or T4) to have metastatic disease at the time of initial presentation.

TNM CLASSIFICATION OF BREAST CANCER

T: Primary Tumor (Figure 3.17)

T1   Tumor 2 cm or less in its greatest dimension
    a. No fixation to underlying pectoral fascia or muscle
    b. Fixation to underlying pectoral fascia or muscle

T2   Tumor more than 2 cm but not more than 5 cm in its greatest dimension

T3   Tumor more than 5 cm in its greatest dimension
    a. No fixation to underlying pectoral fascia or muscle
    b. Fixation to underlying pectoral fascia or muscle

T4   Tumor of any size with direct extension to chest wall or skin
    Note: Chest wall includes ribs, intercostal muscle, and serratus anterior muscle, but not pectoral muscle.
    a. Fixation to chest wall
    b. Edema (including peau d'orange), ulceration of the skin of the breast or satellite skin nodules confined to the same breast
    c. Both of the above
    d. Inflammatory carcinoma

Dimpling of the skin, nipple retraction, or any other skin change except those in T4b may occur in T1, T2, or T3 without affecting the classification.

N: Regional Lymph Nodes

N0   No palpable homolateral axillary nodes

N1   Movable homolateral axillary nodes
    a. Nodes not considered to contain growth
    b. Nodes considered to contain growth

N2   Homolateral axillary nodes containing growth and fixed to one another or to other structures

N3   Homolateral supraclavicular or infraclavicular nodes containing growth or edema of the arm

M: Distant Metastasis

M0   No evidence of distant metastasis

M1   Distant metastasis present, including skin involvement beyond the breast area

TNM STAGING OF BREAST CANCER

Stage I	T1a	N0 or N1a	M0
	T1b	N0 or N1a	
Stage II	T0	N1b	
	T1a	N1b	M0
	T1b	N1b	
	T2a or T2b	N0, N1a, or N1b	
Stage III	T1a or T1b	N2	
	T2a or T2b	N2	M0
	T3a or T3b	N0, N1 or N2	
Stage IV	T4	Any N	M0
	Any T	N3	M0
	Any T	Any N	M1

PATIENT EVALUATION DIAGRAM

See Figure 3.18.

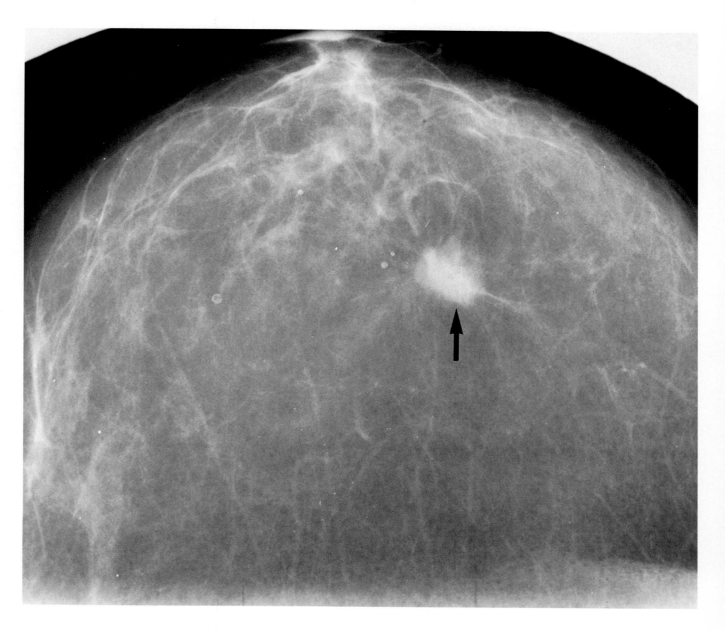

Figure 3.11 Single mammographic view demonstrating infiltrating ductal carcinoma.

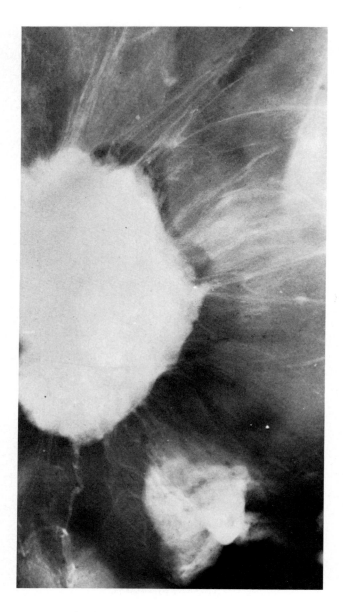

Figure 3.12 *Magnified whole slice specimen radiograph of a large invasive carcinoma showing spiculation of margins, a common radiographic sign of malignancy.*

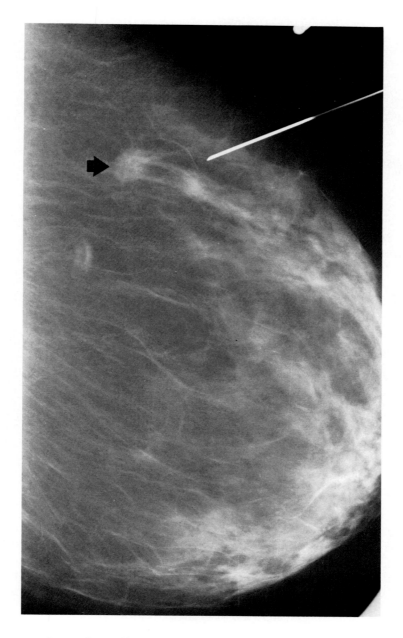

Figure 3.13 *Lateral needle localization mammographic view of a nonpalpable infiltrating ductal carcinoma (arrow).*

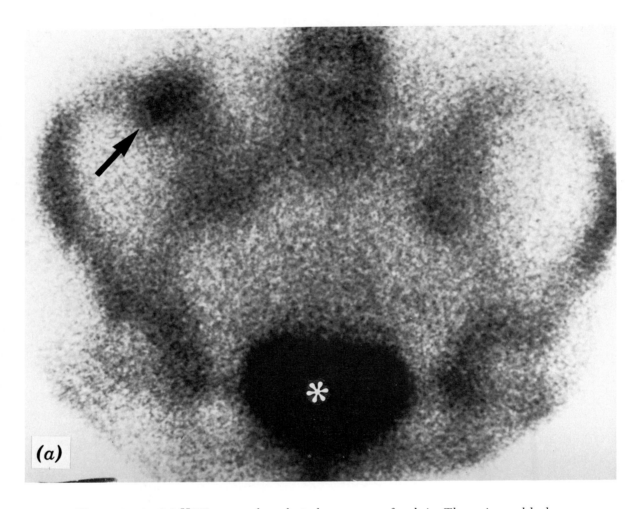

Figure 3.14 (a) ^{99m}Tc-pyrophosphate bone scan of pelvis. The urinary bladder (*) is identified. An area of increased bone activity is present within the right iliac crest (arrow). (b) A plain radiograph of the same pelvis showing the right iliac metastasis (arrow). This lesion was identified only in retrospect after viewing the isotope scan.

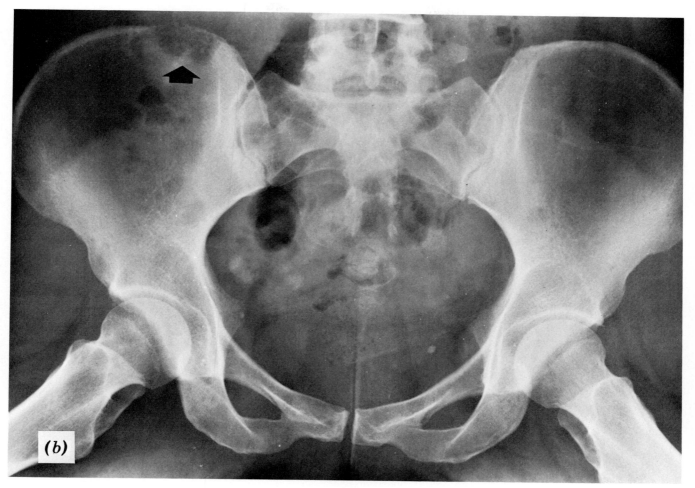

Figure 3.14 (Continued)

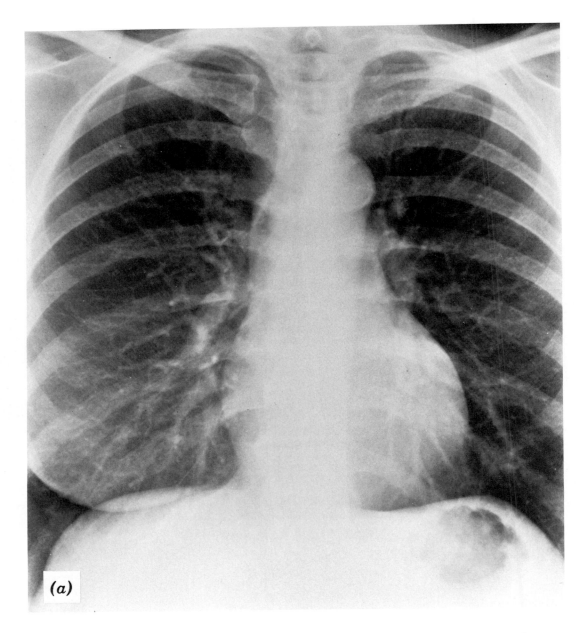

Figure 3.15 (a) Normal chest film of a woman following left mastectomy. (b) Subsequent examination one year later demonstrates right hilar adenopathy (arrow) indicating lymph node metastasis of breast cancer.

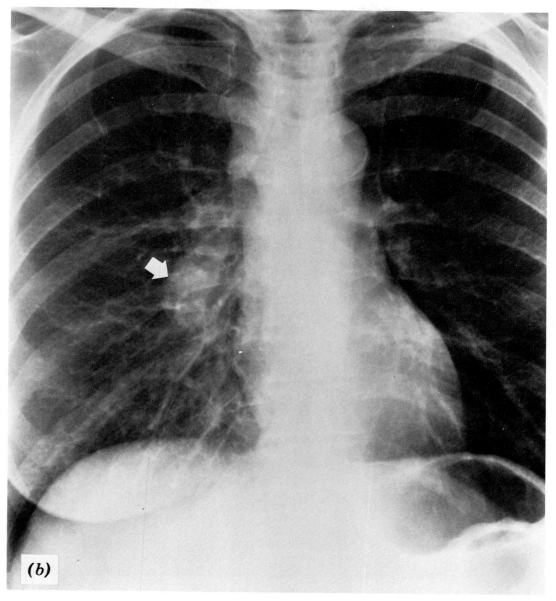

(b)

Figure 3.15 (Continued)

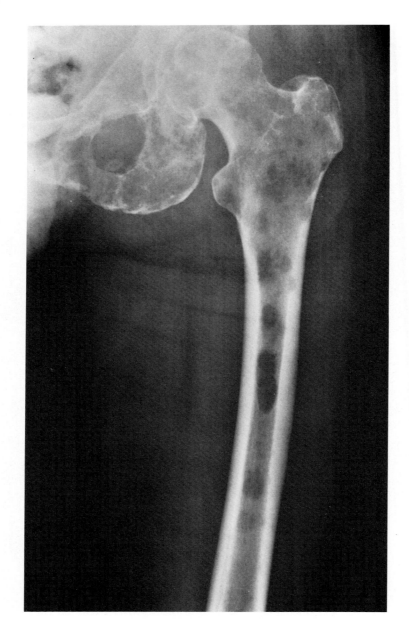

Figure 3.16 Osteolytic metastases in the femoral neck and shaft in a patient with breast cancer.

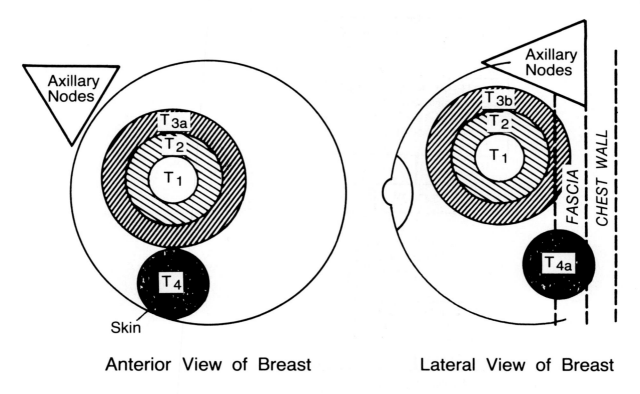

Anterior View of Breast   **Lateral View of Breast**

Figure 3.17 *Schematic diagram of the primary tumor (T) classification of breast cancer.*

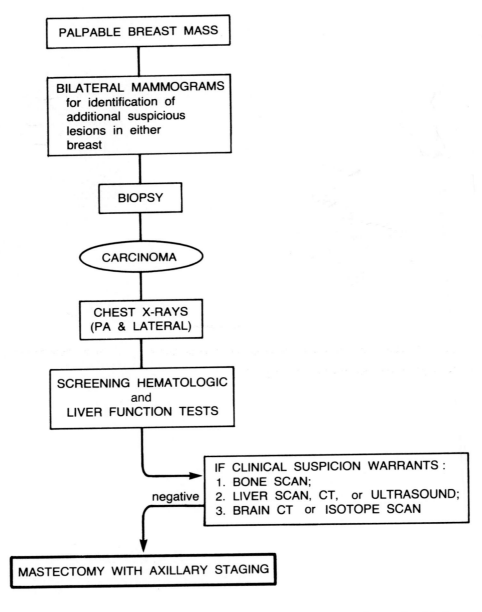

Figure 3.18 *Flow diagram for evaluation of the patient with a palpable breast mass.*

COLORECTAL CANCER

INCIDENCE

126,000 projected new cases in the U.S. in 1983

58,100 deaths

15% of new cancers in Americans

Male:female ratio .94

Colorectal cancer is the second most common cause of cancer deaths in the United States (Figure 3.19).

EPIDEMIOLOGY

The etiology of colon cancer is unknown, but epidemiologic evidence implicates dietary factors. Within the United States high incidence of colorectal cancer is associated with high socioeconomic status and high population density. Worldwide the disease is more common in industrialized than in underdeveloped nations and may be related to dietary fat intake.

A variety of colonic conditions predispose to the development of colorectal cancer: familial colonic polyposis, Gardner's syndrome (colonic polyposis associated with osteomas, fibromas, and lipomas), ulcerative colitis and Crohn's colitis, and villous adenomas. Benign adenomatous polyps, at least in some cases, may undergo malignant degeneration.

PATHOLOGY

The vast majority of colorectal cancers are adenocarcinomas.

TUMOR COMPARTMENT

Tumor Signs and Symptoms

Left Colon and Rectum	Right Colon
Obstructive symptoms (Figure 3.20)	Iron-deficiency anemia (Figure 3.21)
Change in bowel habit	Occult blood in stool
Rectal bleeding, melena	Weight loss
Tenesmus	Weakness
Pain	Cramping pain (late manifestation)
Perforation	Abdominal mass
Change in stool caliber	Perforation
Rectal mass	Asymptomatic

Tumor Diagnosis

Barium enema
Digital rectal examination
Sigmoidoscopy/colonoscopy with biopsy

Tumor Staging

Surgical-pathological staging

LYMPH NODE COMPARTMENT

Lymph Node Signs and Symptoms

Nodal symptoms from colorectal cancer are uncommon.

Lymph Node Staging

Primarily surgical

METASTASIS COMPARTMENT

Metastasis Signs and Symptoms

Liver metastases (Figure 3.22) are most common.

Tender hepatomegaly	Nausea and vomiting
Right upper quadrant discomfort	Jaundice, dark urine
Shoulder pain	Acholic stools
Anorexia and weight loss	Itching

Lung metastases are also frequent but usually asymptomatic.
Distant metastases to other sites are uncommon at the time of diagnosis, but in patients with advanced disease metastases to bone, brain, ovaries, peritoneal surfaces, and other tissues do occur and are common in autopsied patient.

Evaluation for Metastasis

Routine preoperative evaluation for metastatic disease should include careful physical examination with particular attention to the liver, liver function tests, and chest x-ray films (PA and lateral). If these examinations are negative, imaging (including CT, ultrasound, or radionuclide liver scanning) have a very low yield.

On the other hand, if the liver is enlarged to physical examination or if the liver function tests are abnormal, or if the patient has unexplained right upper quadrant symptoms, imaging of the liver is essential.

Modified Dukes Staging System for Colorectal Cancer

A	Confined to mucosa and submucosa
B_1	Penetration into muscularis
B_2	Extension through serosa
C	Regional lymph node involvement
D	Involvement of adjacent organs or distant metastasis

Note: A TNM classification for colorectal cancer exists but is not widely used.

PATIENT EVALUATION DIAGRAM

See Figure 3.23.

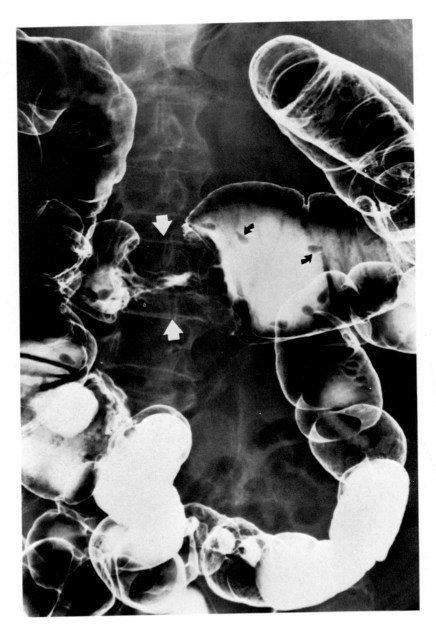

Figure 3.19 Circumferential adenocarcinoma of the midtransverse colon (white arrows). Note ingested grape pits seen in the lumen of the more distal colon (curved arrows).

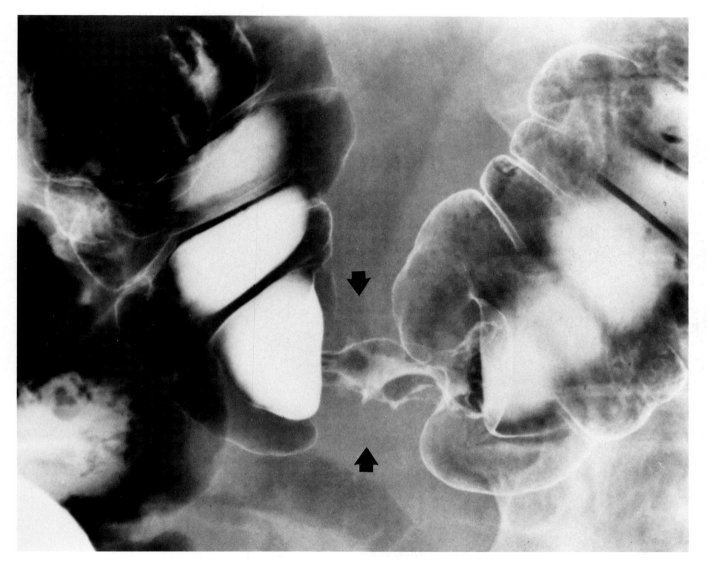

Figure 3.20 Typical "apple-core" appearance of adenocarcinoma of the transverse colon.

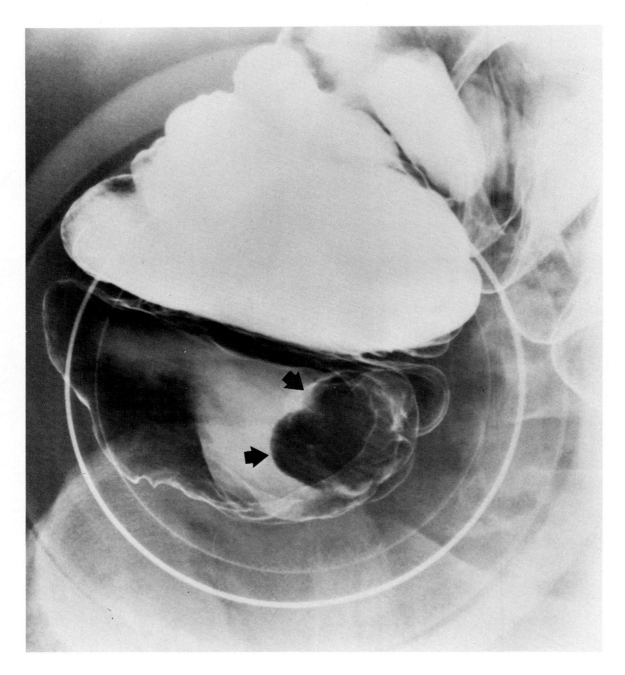

Figure 3.21 *Polypoid adenocarcinoma (arrows) of the cecum.*

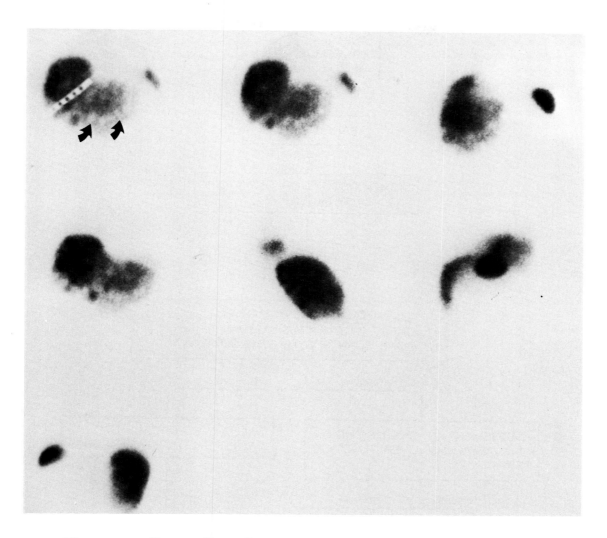

Figure 3.22 ^{99m}Tc-sulfur colloid liver and spleen scan demonstrating multiple focal abnormalities representing metastases (curved arrows).

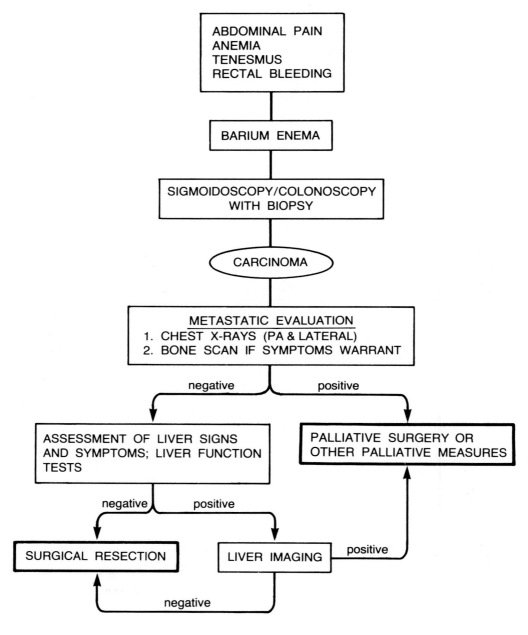

Figure 3.23 *Flow diagram for evaluation of the patient with suspected co-lorectal carcinoma.*

PANCREATIC CANCER

INCIDENCE

25,000 projected new cases in the U.S. in 1983
22,600 deaths
3% of new cancers in Americans
Male:female ratio 1
Fourth most common cause of cancer deaths in the U.S.
Incidence has tripled over the past four decades

EPIDEMIOLOGY

The etiology of pancreatic carcinoma is unknown, but cigarette smoking, diabetes, and certain dietary patterns seem to be associated with increased risk. Blacks are at increased risk for this type of cancer.

PATHOLOGY

Ductal adenocarcinomas: 75%
Other adenocarcinomas (mucinous, acinar, giant cell, adenosquamous, etc): 25%

Seventy percent of pancreatic carcinomas arise within the head of the pancreas, and 20 percent arise in the body and tail. Ten percent involve the pancreas diffusely.

SIGNS AND SYMPTOMS OF PANCREATIC CARCINOMA

	Head	*Body and Tail*
Symptoms:	Weight loss	Weight loss, anorexia
	Jaundice	Abdominal and back pain
	Abdominal and back pain	Weakness
	Anorexia	Nausea and vomiting
	Weakness	Gastrointestinal bleeding
Signs:	Jaundice	Hepatomegaly
	Hepatomegaly	Abdominal mass
	Abdominal mass	Ascites
	Ascites	Jaundice
	Enlarged gallbladder	

DIAGNOSIS AND STAGING OF PANCREATIC CARCINOMA

Ultrasonography (Figure 3.24)

Computerized tomography (Figure 3.25)

Endoscopic retrograde cholangiopancreatography (Figure 3.26)

Percutaneous transhepatic cholangiography (Figure 3.27)

Selective pancreatic angiography (Figure 3.28)—no longer in common use

Tissue diagnosis is made by percutaneous biopsy guided by one of the above imaging techniques.

Surgical staging is also carried out at the time of laparotomy in those patients deemed to have resectable lesions.

METASTASIS COMPARTMENT

Signs and Symptoms

Signs and symptoms of liver metastases

Supraclavicular or other adenopathy

Ascites

Bone pain (uncommon)

Pulmonary signs and symptoms (late manifestation)

Evaluation for Metastasis

At the time of diagnosis most pancreatic carcinomas are unresectable. On occasion, however, a potentially resectable lesion (usually in the head of the pancreas) is encountered. In such cases preoperative evaluation should include careful physical examination with particular attention to liver and lymph node areas, liver function tests, and PA and lateral chest x-ray. The initial CT or ultrasound examination of the pancreas at the time of diagnosis will have included images of the liver, useful in evaluating possible liver metastases preoperatively.

TNM CLASSIFICATION OF PANCREATIC CANCER

T: Primary Tumor

T1 No direct extension of the primary tumor beyond the pancreas

T2 Limited direct extension (to duodenum, bile ducts, or stomach), still possibly permitting tumor resection

T3 Further direct extension, incompatible with surgical resection

TX Direct extension not assessed or not recorded

N: Regional Lymph Nodes

N0   Regional nodes are not involved

N1   Regional nodes involved

NX   Regional node involvement not assessed or not recorded

M: Distant Metastasis

M0   No distant metastasis

M1   Distant metastatic involvement

MX   Distant metastatic involvement not assessed or not recorded

TNM STAGING OF PANCREATIC CANCER

Stage I: T1-2 N0-X M0
              TX N0-X M0

Stage II: T3 N0-X M0

Stage III: T1-3 N1 M0
              TX N1 M0

Stage IV: Any M1

PATIENT EVALUATION DIAGRAM

See Figure 3.29.

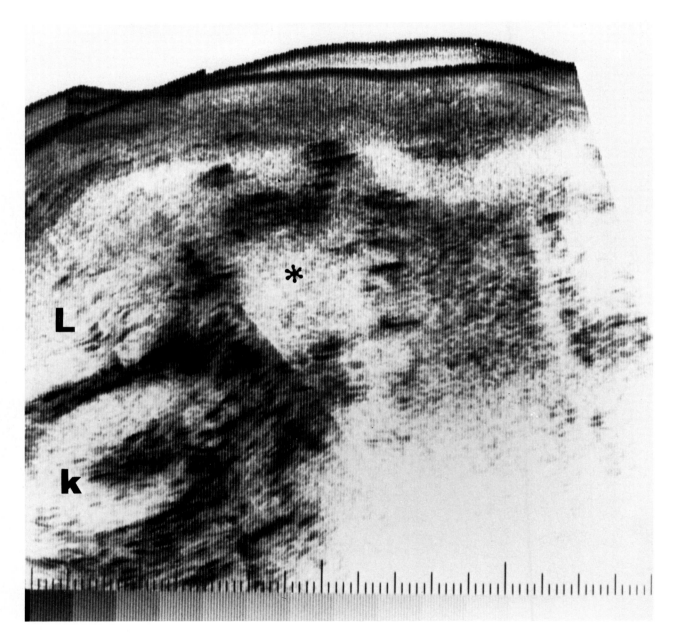

Figure 3.24   Axial ultrasound section of the upper abdomen showing a mass (*) in the head of the pancreas. k, kidney; L, liver.

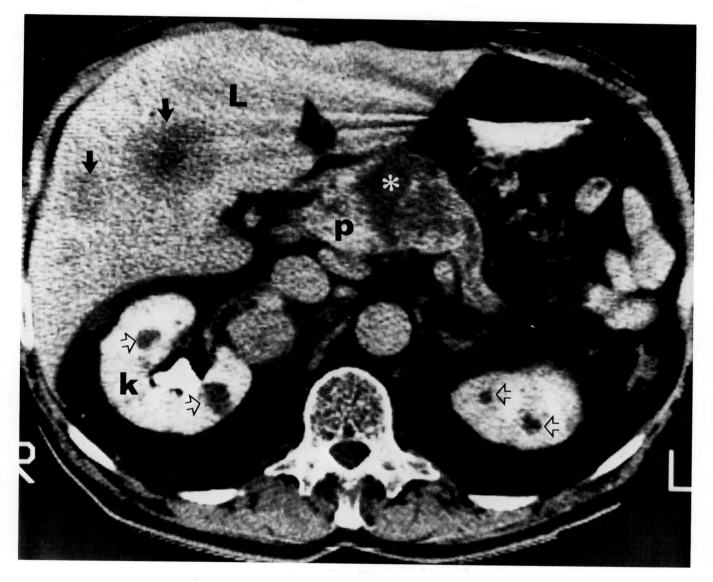

Figure 3.25 Computerized tomogram demonstrating a pancreatic mass (*), hepatic metastases (black arrows), and incidental bilateral simple renal cysts (open arrows). k, kidney; L, liver; p, pancreas.

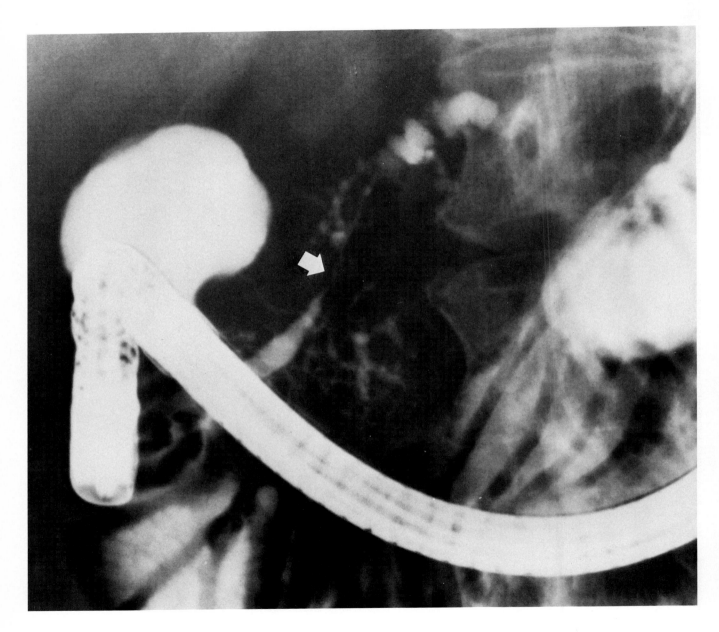

Figure 3.26 *Endoscopic retrograde cholangiopancreatogram demonstrating focal encasement (arrow) of the main pancreatic duct by a pancreatic carcinoma.*

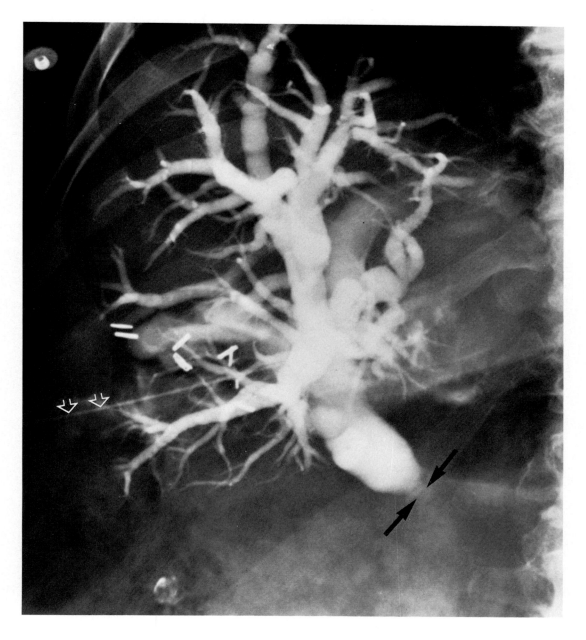

Figure 3.27 Percutaneous transhepatic cholangiogram (PTC) with high grade obstruction (arrows) of the distal common bile duct. Open arrows indicate the Chiba or "skinny" needle used to perform the PTC.

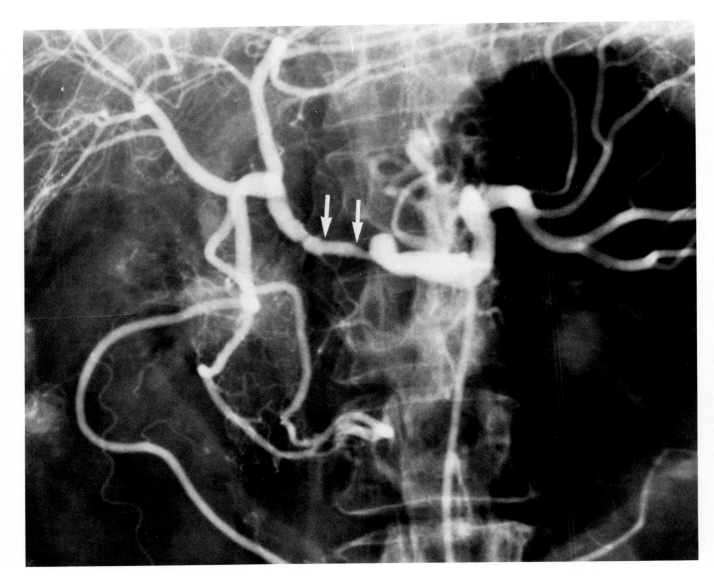

Figure 3.28 *Selective celiac angiogram showing irregular narrowing (encasement) of the common hepatic artery (arrows).*

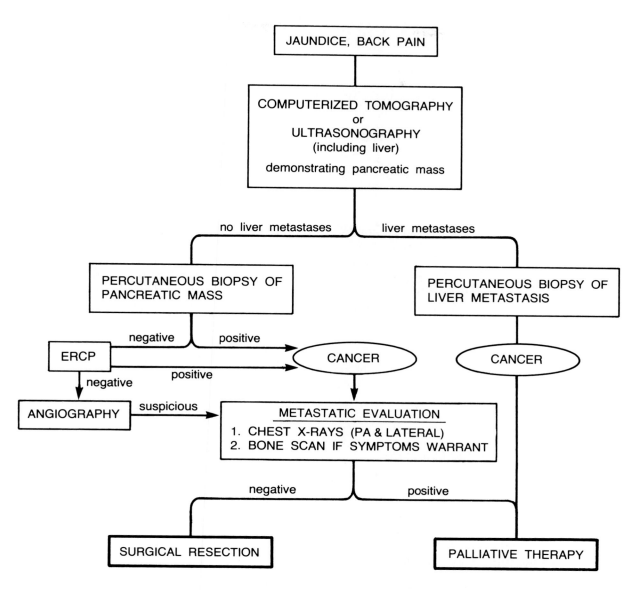

Figure 3.29 *Flow diagram for evaluation of the patient with suspected pancreatic carcinoma.*

GASTRIC CANCER

INCIDENCE

24,500 projected new cases in the U.S. in 1983
13,900 deaths
3% of all new cancers in Americans
Male:female ratio 1
Unexplained marked decrease in incidence in the U.S. over the past 50 years

EPIDEMIOLOGY

Gastric cancer has a wide geographic variation in incidence, with Japan, Chile, Iceland, and Finland having particularly high incidence rates. Numerous dietary substances, including smoked fish, saki, moldy soybean products, and others, have been implicated as possible etiologic factors. Familial occurrence of gastric carcinoma is rare, but there is an increased risk in patients with pernicious anemia and in those with villous adenomas of the stomach.

PATHOLOGY

Ninety-five percent of gastric malignancies are adenocarcinomas. The gross appearance may be polypoid, ulcerating, or infiltrating, which, if extensive, is termed linitis plastica.

TUMOR COMPARTMENT

Tumor Signs and Symptoms

Weight loss	Dysphagia
Epigastric pain	Weakness
Nausea, vomiting	Hematemesis, melena
Anorexia	Epigastric mass

Tumor Diagnosis and Staging

Upper gastrointestinal series (Figure 3.30, 3.31)
Endoscopy with brushing and biopsy

Tumor staging is performed surgically in those patients deemed suitable for gastrectomy.

LYMPH NODE COMPARTMENT

Lymph Node Signs and Symptoms

Nodal involvement due to gastric carcinoma is usually asymptomatic.
Occasionally involvement of the porta hepatis nodes may produce obstructive jaundice.

Lymph Node Staging

Nodal involvement is usually assessed at the time of surgery.
Computerized tomography, often performed to detect liver metastases, may also reveal involvement of perigastric, mesenteric, and para-aortic nodes.

METASTASIS COMPARTMENT

Metastasis Signs and Symptoms

Signs and symptoms of liver metastases
Supraclavicular, axillary, or umbilical adenopathy
Ascites
Bone pain (bone metastases are uncommon)

Pulmonary signs and symptoms are uncommon, but pulmonary metastases are not infrequent.

Evaluation for Metastasis

Although most patients present with locally advanced or widely disseminated disease and are therefore not candidates for curative surgery, in the absence of advanced local disease or distant metastasis surgical resection is indicated. Preoperative evaluation should include careful physical examination with particular attention to liver and lymph nodes, liver function tests, and chest x-ray films. In most cases some form of liver imaging should be performed, even if liver function tests and physical examination are normal, since the detection of clinically occult liver metastases would contraindicate surgery.

TNM CLASSIFICATION OF GASTRIC CANCER

T: Primary Tumor

TX   Degree of penetration of stomach wall not determined
T0   No evidence of primary tumor
T1   Tumor limited to mucosa and submucosa, regardless of its extent or location

T2   Tumor involves the mucosa, the submucosa (including the muscularis propria), and extends to or into the serosa, but does not penetrate through the serosa

T3   Tumor penetrates through the serosa without invading contiguous structures

T4   Tumor penetrates through the serosa and invades the contiguous structures

N: Regional Lymph Nodes

NX   Metastases to intra-abdominal lymph nodes not determined (e.g., laparotomy not done)

N0   No metastases to regional lymph nodes

N1   Involvement of perigastric lymph nodes within 3 cm of the primary tumor along the lesser or greater curvature

N2   Involvement of the regional lymph nodes more than 3 cm from the primary tumor that are removed or removable at operation, including those located along the left gastric, splenic, celiac, and common hepatic arteries

N3   Involvement of other intra-abdominal lymph nodes that are not removable at operation, such as the para-aortic, hepatoduodenal, retropancreatic, and mesenteric nodes

M: Distant Metastasis

MX   Not assessed

M0   No (known) distant metastasis

M1   Distant metastasis present

TNM STAGING OF GASTRIC CANCER

Stage I: T1 N0 M0

Stage II: T2 N0 M0
                T3 N0 M0

Stage III: TX-3 N1-3 M0

Stage IV: T4 NX-3 M0
                Any M1

PATIENT EVALUATION DIAGRAM

See Figure 3.32.

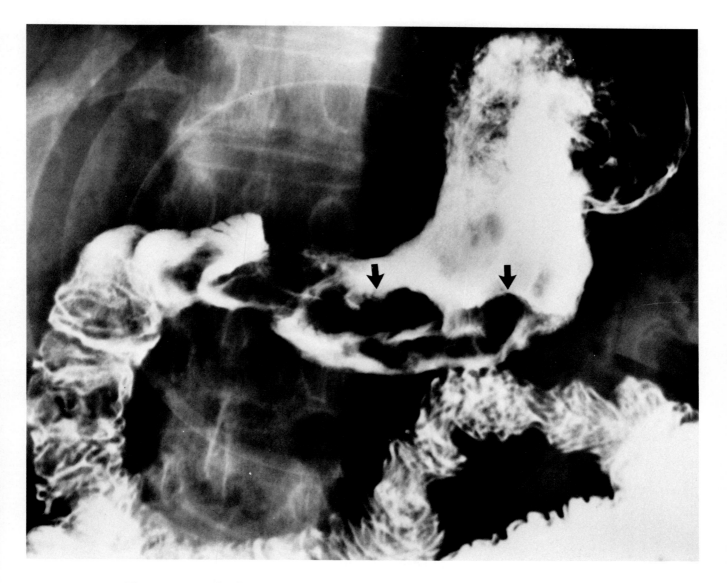

Figure 3.30 Thickened, nodular antral folds (arrows) seen on upper gastrointestinal series. Subsequent gastroscopic biopsy revealed gastric carcinoma.

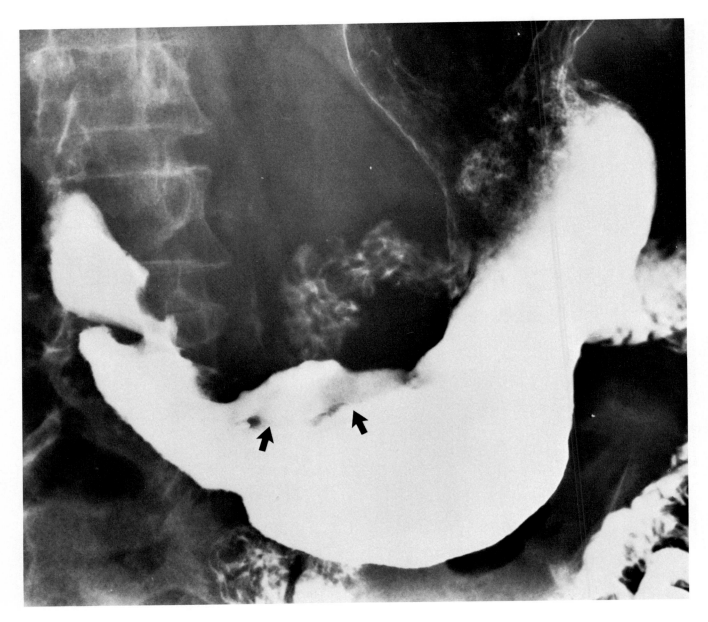

Figure 3.31 Ulcerated gastric carcinoma (arrows).

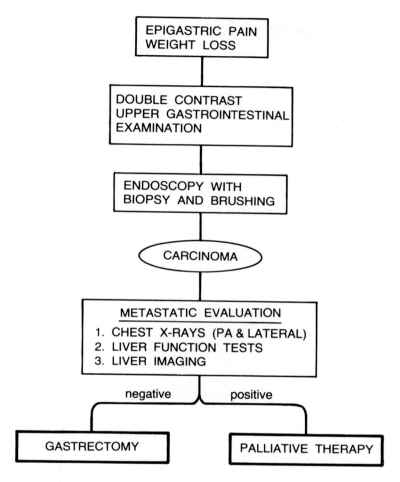

Figure 3.32 *Flow diagram for evaluation of the patient with suspected gastric cancer.*

ESOPHAGEAL CANCER

INCIDENCE

9,000 projected new cases in the U.S. in 1983
8500 deaths
1% of all new cancers in Americans
Male:female ratio 2.5

EPIDEMIOLOGY

There is a wide geographic variation in incidence of esophageal carcinoma; high incidence areas include parts of China, Iran, USSR, Africa, Curacao, and Finland. Certain conditions predispose to esophageal cancer, including alcohol and tobacco use, peptic esophagitis, lye stricture of the esophagus, tylosis palmaris et plantaris, Barrett's esophagus, and Plummer–Vinson syndrome. Esophageal cancer is more than three times as common among American blacks as among whites.

PATHOLOGY

Ninety-eight percent are squamous cell carcinomas and the remaining 2% are adenocarcinomas, which must be distinguished from adenocarcinomas arising in the gastric cardia and extending into the esophagus.

Within the esophagus 50% are located in the lower third (Figure 3.33), 40% in the middle third, and 10% in the upper third.

TUMOR COMPARTMENT

Tumor Signs and Symptoms

Dysphagia
Weight loss
Regurgitation
Vomiting
Pain in throat, substernal or epigastric areas
Aspiration pneumonia
Hematemesis, melena
Persistent cough (tracheoesophageal fistula)

Tumor Diagnosis and Staging

Double contrast barium esophagram (Figure 3.34)
Esophagoscopy with biopsy and brushing
Laryngoscopy and bronchoscopy to detect tumor extension into respiratory tract

LYMPH NODE COMPARTMENT

Lymph Node Signs and Symptoms

Palpable supraclavicular or cervical nodes
Hoarse voice (recurrent laryngeal nerve involvement)
Often asymptomatic

Lymph Node Staging

55° oblique overpenetrated chest film for evaluation of hilar and mediastinal nodes
Computerized tomography of mediastinum and upper abdomen to assess mediastinal and subdiaphragmatic lymph nodes
Mediastinotomy/mediastinoscopy sometimes used to confirm nodal involvement suspected on the basis of imaging procedures

Note: Because esophageal cancer is often locally advanced at the time of diagnosis, only a minority of patients are candidates for curative surgery. Major resections are often performed, nevertheless, for palliative purposes. In these cases, therefore, preoperative lymph node staging would not be necessary since the surgeon could evaluate the lymph nodes during the operation.

METASTASIS COMPARTMENT

Metastasis Signs and Symptoms

Signs and symptoms of liver metastases
Dyspnea due to pleural effusion
Ascites
Bone pain
Diaphragmatic paralysis or hiccups

Evaluation for Metastasis

If surgical palliation or curative surgery is planned, preoperative assessment should include careful physical examination with particular attention to liver and lymph nodes, chest x-ray films, liver function tests, and liver imaging. If the patient is not a surgical candidate, extensive evaluation for distant metastases is unwarranted since local irradiation would be given whether or not metastases were detected.

TNM CLASSIFICATION OF ESOPHAGEAL CANCER

T: Primary Tumor (Figure 3.35)

T0	No demonstrable tumor
TIS	Carcinoma in situ
T1	Tumor involves 5 cm or less or esophageal length with no obstruction nor complete circumferential involvement nor extraesophageal spread
T2	Tumor involves more than 5 cm of esophagus and produces obstruction with circumferential involvement of the esophagus but no extraesophageal spread
T3	Tumor with extension outside the esophagus involving mediastinal structures

N: Regional Lymph Nodes (Figure 3.36)

Cervical esophagus (cervical and supraclavicular lymph nodes):

N0	No nodal involvement
N1	Unilateral involvement (moveable)
N2	Bilateral involvement (moveable)
N3	Fixed nodes

Thoracic esophagus (nodes in the thorax, not those of the cervical, supraclavicular, or abdominal areas):

N0	No nodal involvement
N1	Nodal involvement

M: Distant Metastases

M0	No metastases
M1	Distant metastases. Cancer of thoracic esophagus with cervical, su-

praclavicular, or abdominal lymph node involvement is classified as M1.

TNM STAGING OF ESOPHAGEAL CANCER

Stage I:

T1 N0 M0   Tumor that involves less than 5 cm of esophagus without obstruction and no circumferential nor extraesophageal nor nodal involvement and no metastases

Stage II:

T1 N1 M0   Cervical esophagus: No extraesophageal involvement
T1 N2 M0   with movable regional lymph nodes but no metastases or
T2 N0 M0   a tumor more than 5 cm in size without lymph node in-
T2 N1 M0   volvement
T2 N2 M0

T2 N0 M0   Thoracic esophagus: Any tumor greater than 5 cm in length or producing obstruction or involving the entire circumference of the esophagus without extraesophageal spread

Stage III:

Any M1   Any esophageal cancer with extraesophageal spread or
Any T3   distant metastases

Cervical esophagus: fixed nodes (Any N3).
Thoracic esophagus: regional lymph node involvement (Any N1).

PATIENT EVALUATION DIAGRAM

See Figure 3.37.

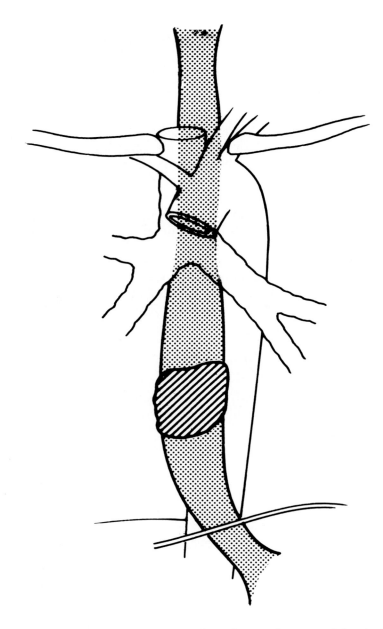

Figure 3.33 *Diagrammatic representation of a carcinoma arising in the distal third of the esophagus, and adjacent anatomic structures.*

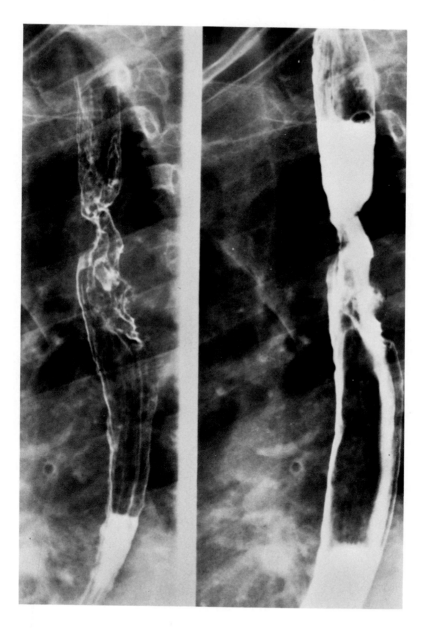

Figure 3.34 Double contrast esophagram showing a circumferential (T2) midesophageal carcinoma.

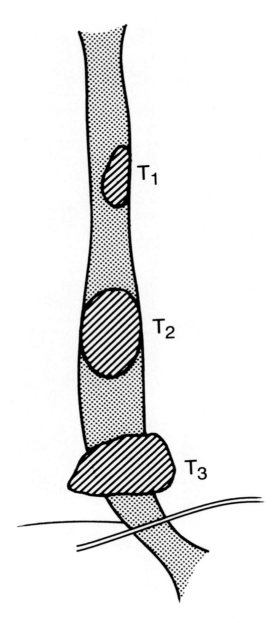

Figure 3.35 *Primary tumor (T) classification of esophageal carcinoma.*

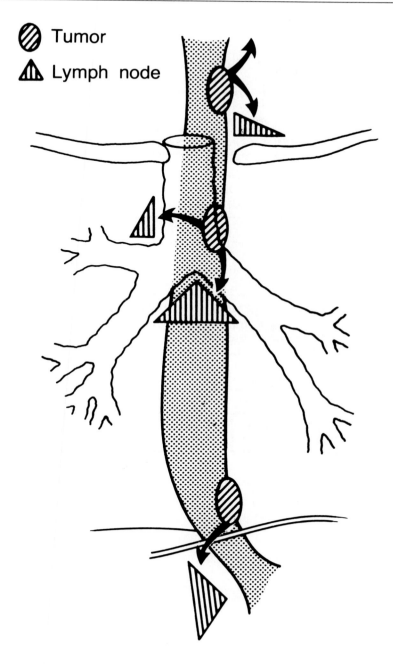

Figure 3.36 Regional lymph node metastases of esophageal carcinoma. Note that lymphatic spread is dependent upon the site of the primary lesion.

139

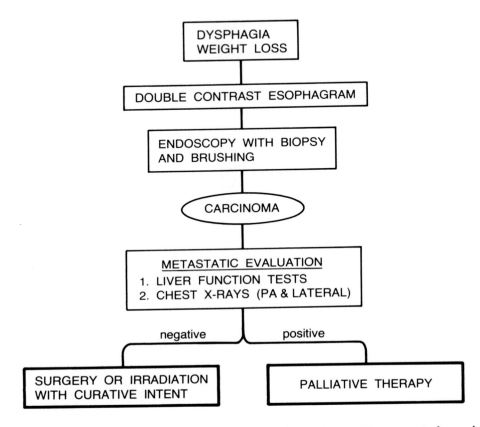

Figure 3.37 *Flow diagram for evaluation of the patient with suspected esophageal cancer.*

HEPATOBILIARY CANCER

INCIDENCE

13,300 projected new cases in the U.S. in 1983
10,000 deaths
1.6% of all new cancers in Americans
Male:female ratio .9

Gallbladder cancer, like benign gallbladder disease, is more common in women.

EPIDEMIOLOGY

Hepatoma: Several carcinogens have been implicated in the etiology of hepatoma, including aflatoxin, *Senecio* alkaloids from certain plants, and steroid hormones (androgens, birth control pills). Also, vinyl chloride exposure predisposes to the extremely rare hepatic angiosarcoma. Hepatomas are much more common in the Far East and South Africa. In the United States most hepatomas arise in cirrhotic livers. About 5% of cirrhotics develop hepatoma. There is an association between hepatitis B antigenemia and hepatoma as well.

Gallbladder cancer: Most cases (65–90%) of gallbladder cancer arise in patients with cholelithiasis. However, only 2% of surgically removed gallbladders contain carcinoma. Patients with porcelain gallbladders are at high risk for gallbladder cancer. American Indians of the Southwest are also a high-risk population.

Bile duct cancer: American Indians have an increased incidence of primary biliary tract cancer, as do patients with *Clonorchis sinensis* infestation and ulcerative colitis. There appears to be no relationship between cholelithiasis and bile duct cancer, however.

PATHOLOGY

The majority of hepatobiliary malignancies are adenocarcinomas, but squamous cell carcinomas of the gallbladder and bile ducts do occur. Angiosarcoma of the liver, an extremely rare tumor, is virtually limited to patients with an occupational exposure to vinyl chloride.

HEPATOMA

Signs and Symptoms

Rapid deterioration in a patient with cirrhosis, i.e., jaundice, increased ascites, abdominal pain, cachexia, fever, increasing hepatomegaly

In a patient without cirrhosis, right upper quadrant pain and mass, fever, Budd–Chiari syndrome, intraperitoneal hemorrhage

Hypoglycemia

Hypercalcemia

Polycythemia

Hepatic friction rub

Diagnosis and Staging

Computerized tomography (Figure 3.38)

Ultrasonography

Alpha-fetoprotein; useful if positive, but neither completely specific nor highly sensitive

Biopsy via percutaneous, peritoneoscopic, or surgical routes

Angiography (Figure 3.39) for preoperative mapping

No TNM or other staging system is in use

PATIENT EVALUATION DIAGRAM

See Figure 3.40.

GALLBLADDER CANCER

Signs and Symptoms

Most signs and symptoms of gallbladder cancer are the same as those associated with benign gallbladder disease: right upper quandrant pain, anorexia, nausea, vomiting, obstructive jaundice, weight loss, right upper quadrant mass.

Diagnosis and Staging

In most cases the diagnosis of gallbladder cancer is not suspected preoperatively, and the tumor is an unanticipated finding at surgery for presumed benign gallbladder disease. Laboratory and imaging evaluations are not useful for distinguishing benign from malignant gallbladder disease. No TNM or other staging system for this tumor is available.

BILE DUCT CANCER

Signs and Symptoms

Obstructive jaundice   Weight loss, anorexia, nausea
Pruritus   Hepatomegaly
Right upper quadrant pain   Palpable gallbladder

Diagnosis and Staging

Ultrasonography (Figure 3.41) or computerized tomography (Figure 3.42) to confirm biliary obstruction

Endoscopic retrograde cholangiopancreatography (Figure 3.43)

Percutaneous transhepatic cholangiography

Percutaneous biopsy guided by PTC or ERCP, or surgical exploration with biopsy and resection or palliative biliary diversion

No TNM or other staging system for this tumor is available

PATIENT EVALUATION DIAGRAM

See Figure 3.44.

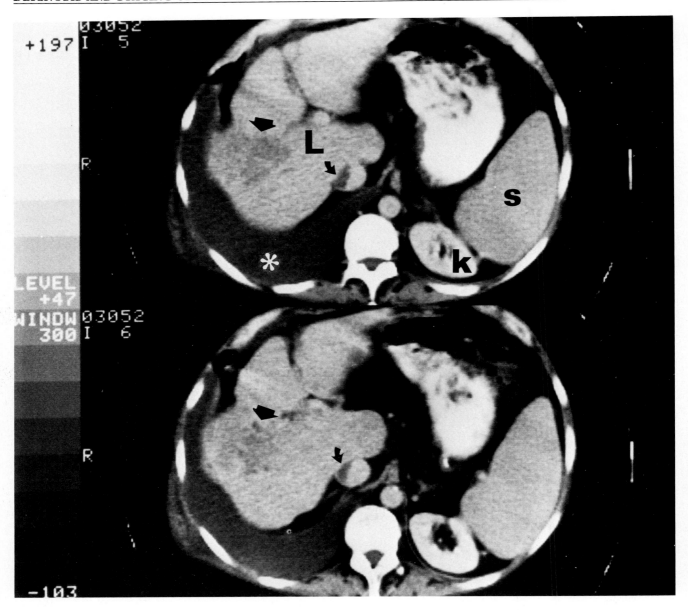

Figure 3.38 *Computerized tomographic sections through the upper abdomen demonstrating an inhomogeneous hepatic tumor (arrow heads) within a deformed and nodular cirrhotic liver. A tumor thrombus (curved arrows) is seen within the inferior vena cava. A right pleural effusion (*) is present. The diagnosis of hepatoma was made at autopsy L, liver; k, kidney; S, spleen.*

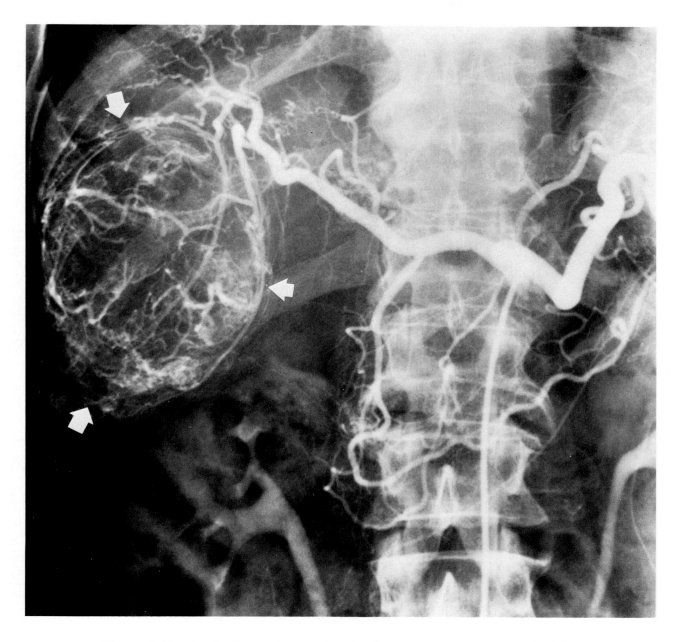

Figure 3.39 *A selective celiac angiogram demonstrates a circumscribed hepatic tumor (arrows) with abnormal vessels (neovascularity). A diagnosis of hepatoma was confirmed by biopsy.*

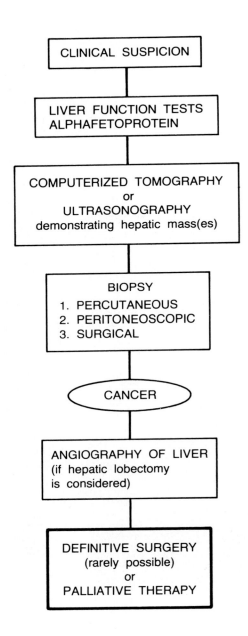

Figure 3.40 *Flow diagram for evaluation of the patient with suspected hepatoma.*

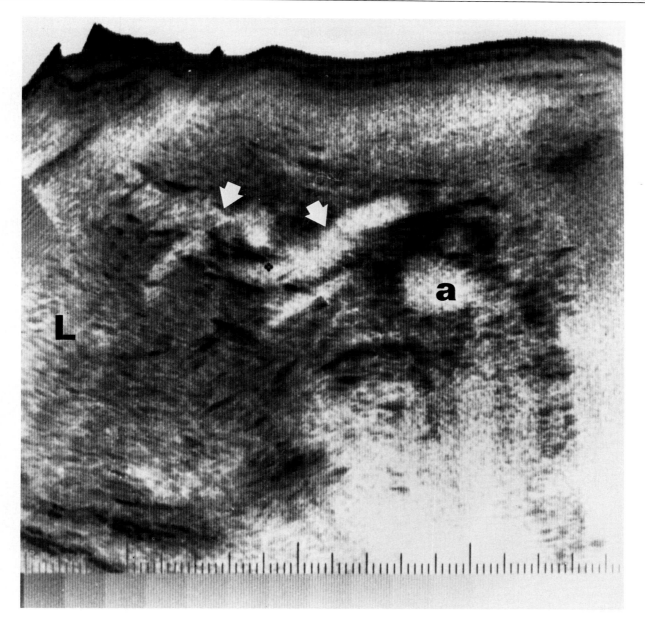

Figure 3.41 *Transverse ultrasound section through the upper abdomen demonstrating dilated intrahepatic biliary ducts (arrows). The liver (L) and aorta (a) are identified. Subsequent PTC with percutaneous biopsy verified the diagnosis of primary bile duct carcinoma.*

147

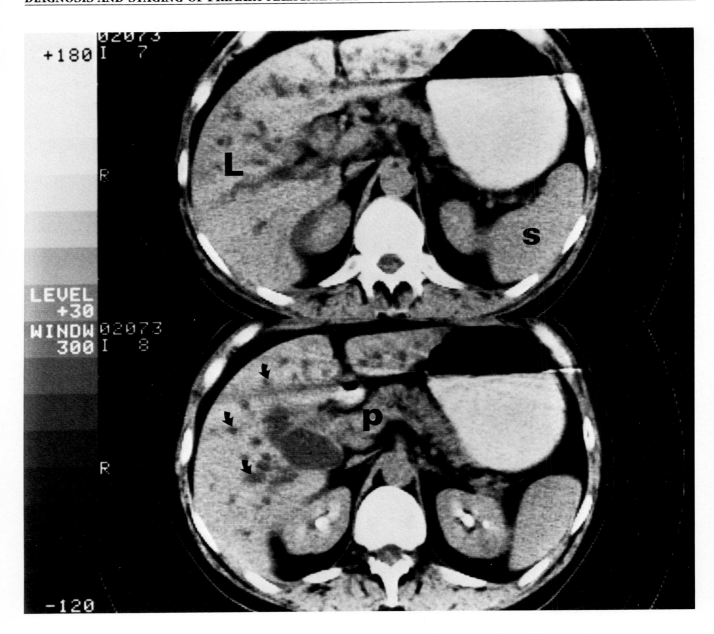

Figure 3.42 *Computerized tomographic sections through a liver (L) containing obstructed biliary radicles (arrows). The pancreas (P) and spleen (s) are
normal. Subsequent PTC and percutaneous biopsy demonstrated a primary
carcinoma of the common hepatic duct.*

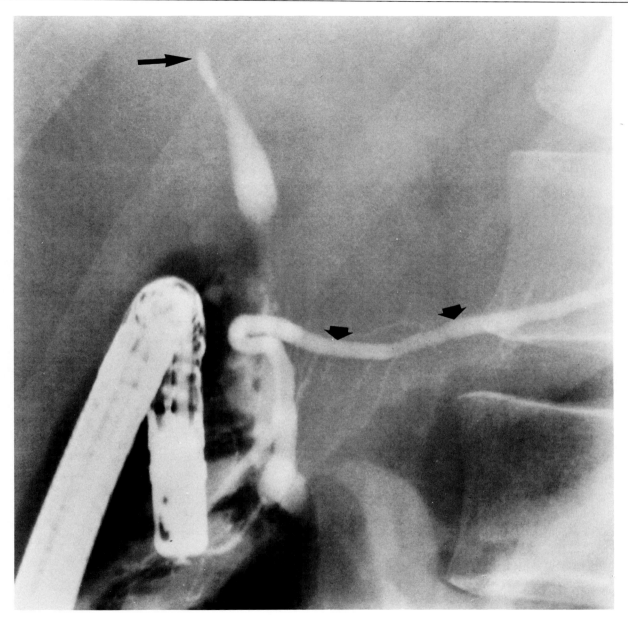

Figure 3.43 *Endoscopic retrograde cholangiopancreatogram showing a normal pancreatic duct (arrow heads) and a proximally obstructed common bile duct (long arrow). Exploratory surgery revealed a cholangiocarcinoma arising in the proximal common bile duct.*

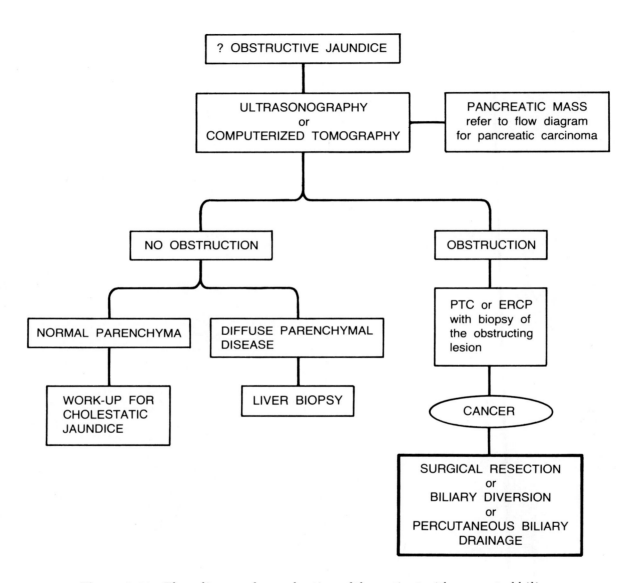

Figure 3.44 *Flow diagram for evaluation of the patient with suspected biliary tract cancer.*

SMALL BOWEL CANCER

INCIDENCE

2,100 projected new cases in the U.S. in 1983
700 deaths
Male:female ratio 1.0
1% of all gastrointestinal malignancies

EPIDEMIOLOGY

Predisposing conditions include Peutz-Jeghers syndrome and von Recklinghausen's neurofibromatosis.

PATHOLOGY

Approximately 50% of small bowel malignancies are adenocarcinomas, occurring most often in the proximal jejunum and duodenum. Carcinoid tumors are next most frequent and arise predominantly in the terminal ileum. Leiomyosarcomas, lymphomas, and other soft tissue sarcomas comprise most of the remaining small bowel malignancies.

Metastatic tumors are rare and may include melanoma, breast cancer, and lung cancer. Obviously the small bowel may be involved by direct extension from tumors of the colon, stomach, kidney, genitourinary tract, and other sites.

TUMOR COMPARTMENT

Tumor Signs and Symptoms

Abdominal pain
Weight loss
Intestinal obstruction
Intestinal bleeding
Diarrhea (particularly with lymphomas)
Jaundice (with periampullary carcinomas)
Palpable abdominal mass
Carcinoid syndrome (usually requires liver metastases)

151

Tumor Diagnosis and Staging

    Upper gastrointestinal series with small bowel follow-through (Figure 3.45)

    Barium enema for tumor of the terminal ileum

    Small bowel endoscopy and biopsy (rarely possible beyond ligament of Treitz)

    ERCP for duodenal and ampullary tumors

    Abdominal angiography for patients who present with intestinal hemorrhage

LYMPH NODE COMPARTMENT

Signs and symptoms due to lymph node involvement with small intestinal cancers are very rare. Lymph node staging is entirely surgical.

METASTASIS COMPARTMENT

Distant metastases (Figure 3.46) from small bowel malignancies may involve lung, liver, bone, and other sites less commonly. In most cases, however, surgical treatment is necessary to relieve the symptoms caused by the primary lesion, whether or not metastases are present. Therefore, the presurgical evaluation for distant metastases in most cases requires only a careful physical examination, chest x-ray films, and liver function tests.

No TNM or other staging system for small bowel cancers is available.

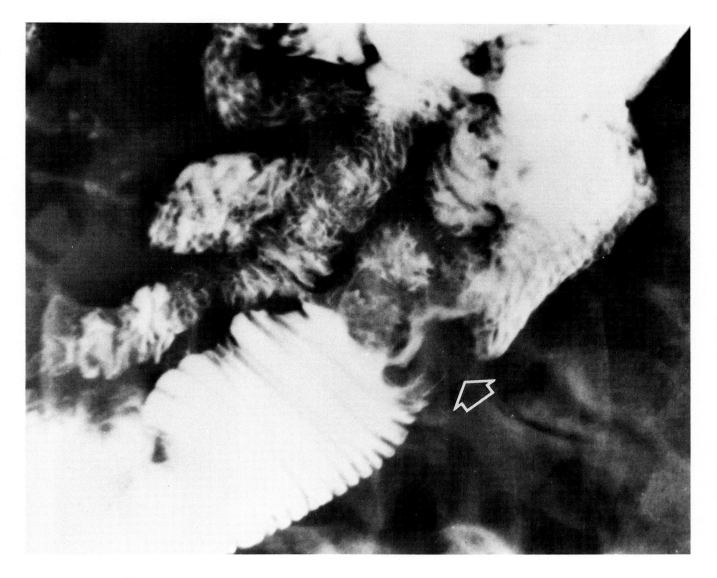

Figure 3.45 *Eccentric mass in the jejunum (arrow) representing a primary small bowel adenocarcinoma.*

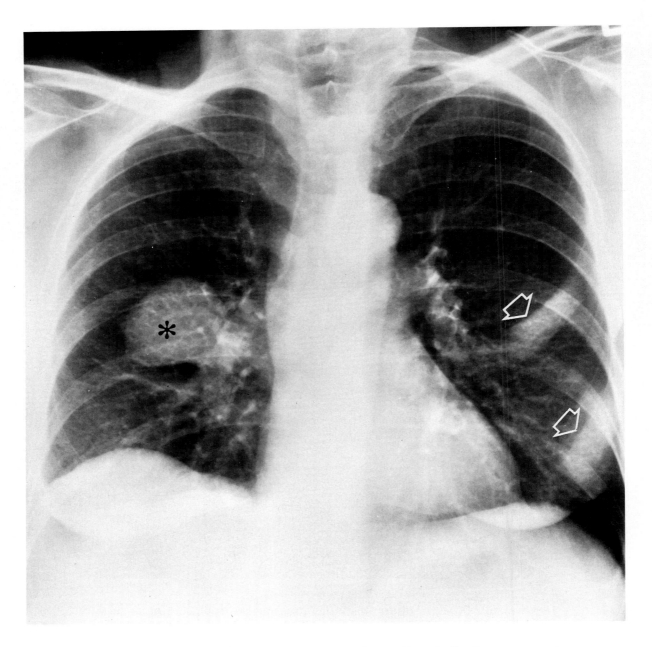

Figure 3.46 *Carcinoid tumor metastatic to lung (*) and ribs (open arrows). Osteoblastic lesions are typical of metastatic carcinoid.*

RENAL CELL CARCINOMA

INCIDENCE

18,200 projected new cases in the U.S. in 1983
8,500 deaths
2% of all new cancers in Americans
Male:female ratio 1.7

EPIDEMIOLOGY

The etiology of renal cell carcinoma is unknown (Figure 3.47), but epidemiologic studies have shown an increased incidence among tobacco users and in patients exposed to thorotrast, an obsolete radiologic contrast agent.

PATHOLOGY

Eighty-five percent of renal cancers are adenocarcinomas. The remainder are mostly transitional cell carcinomas originating in the collecting system.

TUMOR COMPARTMENT

Tumor Signs and Symptoms

Hematuria	Fever
Flank pain	Anemia
Abdominal mass	Erythrocytosis
Weight loss	Hypercalcemia
Hypertension	Acute varicocele

Tumor Diagnosis and Staging

Excretory urography with nephrotomography (Figure 3.48): initial examination for most patients with hematuria. Useful in distinguishing solid from cystic renal masses with high reliability.

Computerized tomography (Figure 3.49): confirms solid nature of masses seen on urography. Defines extrarenal extension of tumor and may upgrade a T2 lesion to T3 or T4.

Ultrasonography: an alternative to computerized tomography for assessing solid nature of renal masses but less reliable for defining tumor extent.

Renal angiography: useful for surgical planning but not required for diagnostic and staging evaluation.

Inferior vena cavography (Figure 3.50): helpful in planning technical details of surgical approach, and may upgrade a T1 or T2 lesion to a T3 or T4.

LYMPH NODE COMPARTMENT

Lymph Node Signs and Symptoms

Usually asymptomatic

Lower extremity edema due to extrinsic nodal compression of inferior vena cava (rare)

Respiratory distress due to mediastinal nodal involvement (rare)

Lymph Node Staging

Computerized tomography

In most cases nodal staging is accomplished at the time of surgery

METASTASIS COMPARTMENT

In cases in which curative surgery is contemplated, assessment of the metastatic compartment should include, in addition to physical examination, chest x-ray films, liver function tests, and liver imaging. (Computerized tomography, ultrasonography, and angiography, if already performed for tumor evaluation, should be reviewed for the possible presence of liver metastases). Any clinical indication of bone or brain metastasis should be followed by appropriate imaging of those sites. Although the diagnostic yield of whole lung plain film or computerized tomography is low in the face of a normal chest x-ray film, these studies may detect occult pulmonary nodules, the presence of which would render curative surgery inappropriate.

Ten percent of patients with renal cell carcinoma present with manifestations of metastatic disease while harboring a clinically silent renal primary. Biopsy of the metastatic site often suggests a carcinoma of renal origin.

TNM CLASSIFICATION OF RENAL CELL CARCINOMA

T: Primary Tumor (Figure 3.51)

T0   No evidence of primary tumor

T1   Small tumor, minimal renal and calyceal distortion or deformity. Circumscribed neovasculature surrounded by normal parenchyma

T2	Large tumor with deformity and/or enlargement of kidney and/or collecting system
T3a	Tumor involving perinephric tissues
T3b	Tumor involving renal vein
T3c	Tumor involving renal vein and infradiaphragmatic vena cava
T4a	Tumor invasion of neighboring structures (e.g., muscle, bowel)
T4b	Tumor involving supradiaphragmatic vena cava

N: Regional Lymph Nodes (Figure 3.52)

The regional lymph nodes are the para-aortic and paracaval nodes. The juxtaregional lymph nodes are the pelvic nodes and the mediastinal nodes.

N0	No evidence of involvement of regional nodes
N1	Single, homolateral regional nodal involvement
N2	Involvement of multiple regional or contralateral or bilateral nodes
N3	Fixed regional nodes (assessable only at surgical exploration)
N4	Involvement of juxtaregional nodes

M: Distant Metastasis

MX	Not assessed
M0	No (known) distant metastasis
M1	Distant metastasis present

STAGING SYSTEM FOR RENAL CELL CARCINOMA (Figure 3.53)

Stage I:	Tumor confined to the kidney
Stage II:	Tumor locally invasive but confined to Gerota's fascia
Stage III:	Regional invasion
	A. Invasion of renal vein or vena cava or both
	B. Metastases to regional lymph nodes
	C. Combination of A and B
Stage IV:	A. Invasion of surrounding organs (other than adrenal glands)
	B. Distant metastases

PATIENT EVALUATION DIAGRAM

See Figure 3.54.

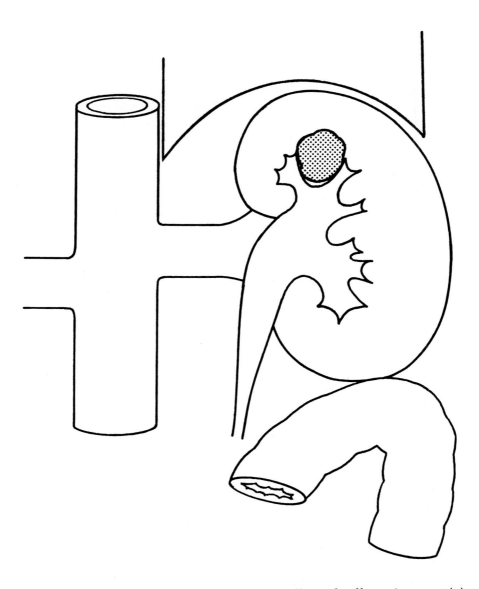

Figure 3.47 *Schematic representation of a small renal cell carcinoma arising in the upper pole of the left kidney.*

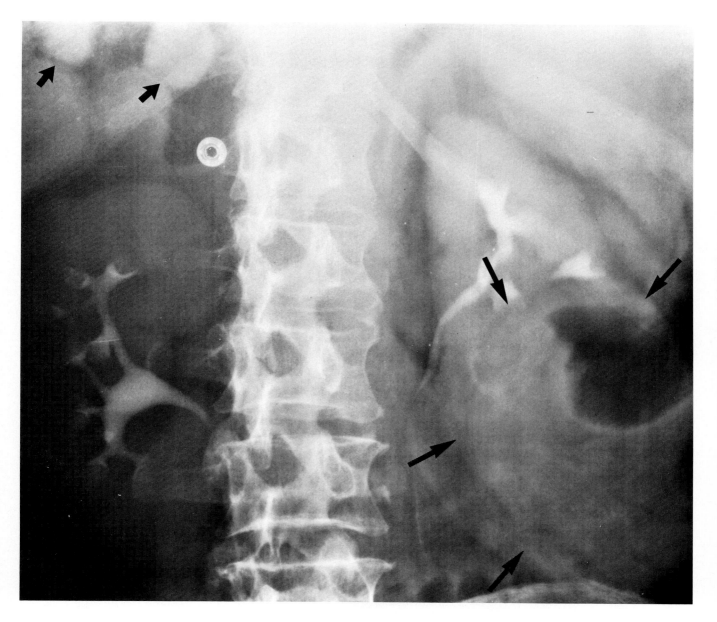

Figure 3.48 Excretory urogram demonstrating left lower pole renal mass (long arrows). Note pulmonary metastases (short arrows).

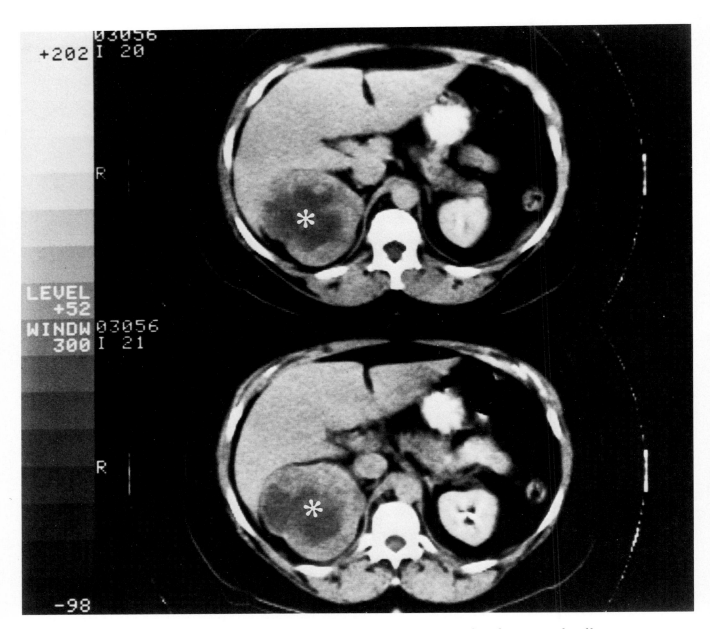

Figure 3.49 *Computerized tomographic sections through a large renal cell carcinoma (*). The liver as seen in these sections appears normal.*

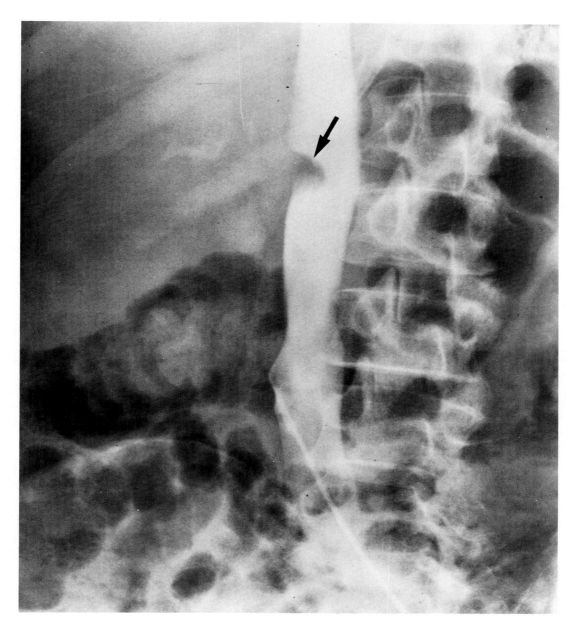

Figure 3.50 *Inferior vena cavagram with tumor thrombus (arrow) extending from the right renal vein in a patient with renal cell carinoma.*

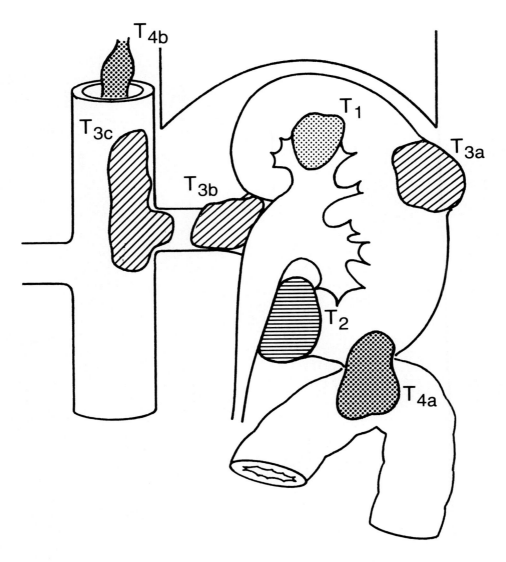

Figure 3.51 *Primary tumor (T) classification of renal cell carcinoma.*

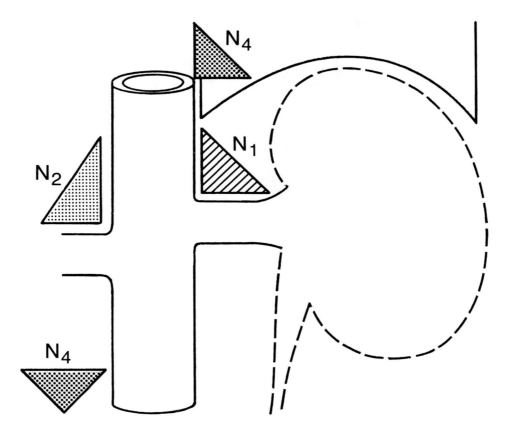

Figure 3.52 *Regional lymph node (N) classification of renal cell carcinoma. N3 (fixed regional nodes) is not shown since it can only be assessed at surgery. N4 represents either a mediastinal or a pelvic lymph node.*

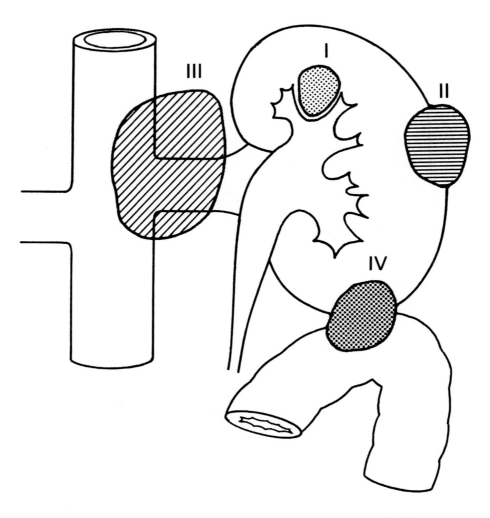

Figure 3.53 *Schematic diagram of the staging system for renal cell carcinoma.*

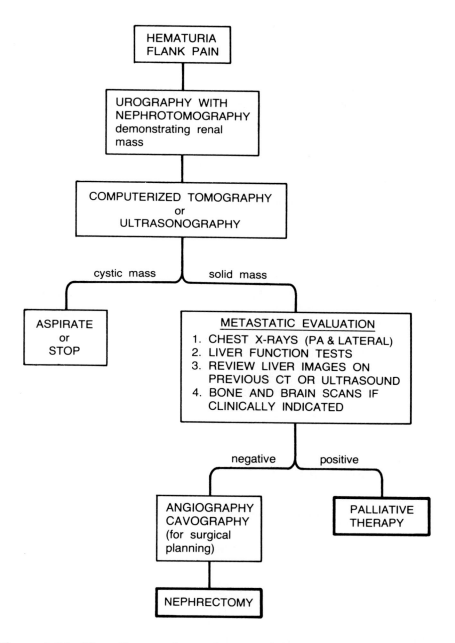

Figure 3.54 *Flow diagram for evaluation of the patient with suspected renal cell carcinoma. Note: A tissue diagnosis of malignancy is usually not obtained before nephrectomy in those patients who are surgical candidates. In patients with metastatic disease, tissue diagnosis is usually made by percutaneous biopsy of a metastatic lesion (often in liver or lung).*

BLADDER CANCER

INCIDENCE

38,500 projected new cases in the U.S. in 1983
10,700 deaths
4.5% of new cancers in Americans
Male:female ratio 2.7

EPIDEMIOLOGY

Increased risk of bladder cancer is associated with bladder schistosomiasis, cigarette smoking, and occupational exposure to certain aromatic amines (such as those found in the aniline dye industry and the plastics industry).

PATHOLOGY

Over 98% of bladder cancers are transitional cell carcinomas; 6–8% are squamous cell carcinomas, and the remainder are adenocarcinomas. Tumor stage and prognosis are related to tumor grade.

TUMOR COMPARTMENT

Tumor Signs and Symptoms

Hematuria	Dysuria
Suprapubic pain	Acute urinary retention
Urinary frequency	Urinary tract infection

Tumor Diagnosis and Staging

Excretory urography (Figure 3.55): initial imaging procedure in patients with hematuria. Also used to assess the presence and degree of ureteral obstruction
Urinary cytology
Cystoscopy with biopsy
Bimanual examination under anesthesia
Computerized tomography of pelvis (Figure 3.56); may upgrade to a T4

LYMPH NODE COMPARTMENT

Lymph Node Signs and Symptoms

Usually asymptomatic
Palpable inguinal adenopathy

Lymph Node Diagnosis and Staging

Lymphography: greater sensitivity than computerized tomography
Computerized tomography: detects bulky lymph node disease
Surgical staging

METASTASIS COMPARTMENT

When radical cystectomy is planned, preoperative evaluation, for distant metastasis should include careful physical examination, chest x-ray films, liver function tests, and probably radionuclide bone scan, since the incidence of bone metastases at the time of diagnosis seems to be higher than previously recognized.

TNM CLASSIFICATION OF BLADDER CANCER

T: Primary Tumor

T0   No evidence of primary tumor

TIS   Sessile carcinoma in situ

Ta   Papillary noninvasive carcinoma

T1   On bimanual examination a freely mobile mass may be felt; this should not be felt after complete transurethral resection of the lesion and/or there is papillary carcinoma without microscopic invasion beyond the lamina propria

T2   On bimanual examination there is induration of the bladder wall, which is mobile; there is no residual induration after complete transurethral resection of the lesion and/or there is microscopic invasion of superfical muscle of bladder

T3   On bimanual examination there is induration or a nodular mobile mass is palpable in the bladder wall that persists after transurethral resection

T3a   Microscopic invasion of deep muscle

T3b   Invasion through the full thickness of bladder wall

T4   Tumor fixed or invading neighboring structures and/or there is microscopic evidence of invasion of the prostate and in the other circumstances listed below at least muscle invasion

T4a   Tumor invading substance of prostate, uterus, or vagina

T4b   Tumor fixed to the pelvic wall and/or infiltrating the abdominal wall

N: Regional Lymph Nodes

The regional lymph nodes are the pelvic nodes just below the bifurcation of the common iliac arteries. The juxtaregional lymph nodes are the inguinal nodes, the common iliac, and para-aortic nodes.

N0   No involvement of regional lymph nodes

N1   Involvement of a single homolateral regional lymph node

N2   Involvement of contralateral, bilateral, or multiple regional lymph nodes

N3   There is a fixed mass on the pelvic wall with a free space between it and the tumor

N4   Involvement of juxtaregional lymph nodes

M: Distant Metastasis

MX   Not assessed

M0   No (known) distant metastasis

M1   Distant metastasis present

STAGING SYSTEM FOR BLADDER CANCER

Several overlapping, competing staging systems for bladder cancer are in current use, making this a very confusing area. Use of the TNM system will reduce this confusion.

Jewett-Marshall System	TNM System	Description
Stage 0	TIS	Carcinoma in situ
Stage A	T1	Subepithelial invasion
Stage B1	T2	Superficial muscle invasion
Stage B2, C	T3	Deep muscle invasion
Stage D	T4	Invasion of adjacent organs
Stage D1	N1–3	Involvement of regional nodes
Stage D2	N4	Involvement of juxtaregional nodes

PATIENT EVALUATION DIAGRAM

See Figure 3.57.

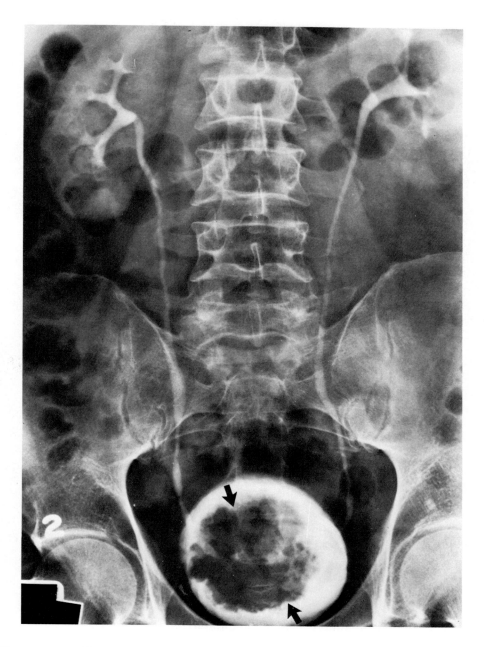

Figure 3.55 *Excretory urogram showing a large bladder tumor (arrows).*

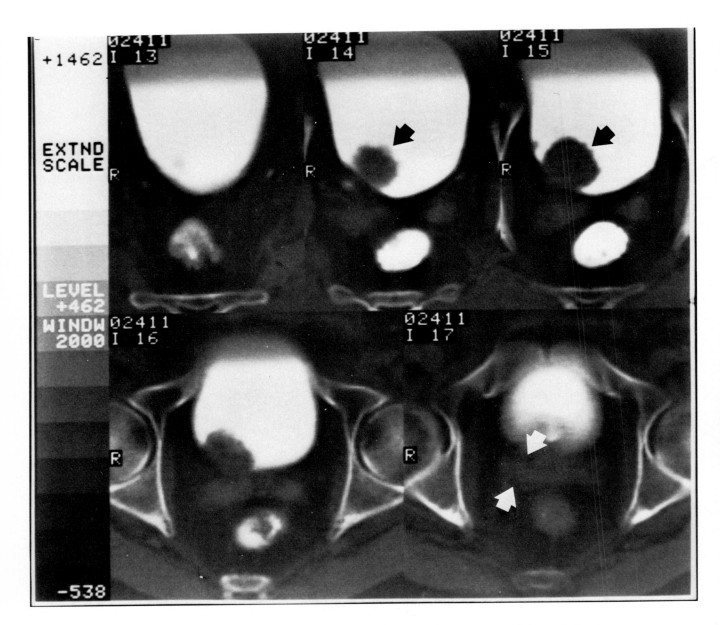

Figure 3.56 *Multiple images from a computerized tomogram of the pelvis. A tumor is seen within the contrast-filled bladder (black arrow). The right seminal vesicle is thickened and presumed to be involved with tumor (white arrows).*

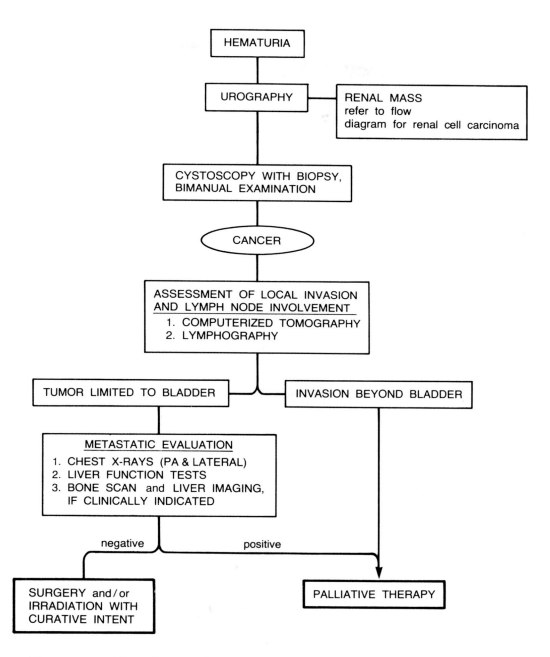

Figure 3.57 *Flow diagram for evaluation of the patient with suspected bladder cancer.*

171

PROSTATE CANCER

INCIDENCE

75,000 projected new cases in the U.S. in 1983 (Figure 3.58)

24,100 deaths

8.7% of new cancers in Americans

18% of new cancers in American males

Second most common cause of cancer deaths in American males

Incidence rises rapidly with increasing age, peaking in the seventh and eighth decades

Microscopic prostatic carcinoma is found in routine autopsy specimens in 15–20% of men in their fifties and 60% of men in their eighties

EPIDEMIOLOGY

The etiology of prostate cancer is unknown. American blacks have the world's highest incidence, Japanese have among the lowest. Marked geographic variation in incidence rates worldwide is observed. No carcinogens for prostate cancer have been identified, but a hormonal effect is recognized: castrated men and those with hyperestrogenism do not develop prostate cancer.

PATHOLOGY

More than 95% of prostate cancers are adenocarcinomas.

TUMOR COMPARTMENT

Tumor Signs and Symptoms

Many prostate cancers are asymptomatic and are detected by palpation of a prostatic nodule on routine digital rectal examination.

Urinary frequency

Difficulty initiating micturition

Urinary retention

Hematuria

Tissue Diagnosis

Transrectal or transperineal needle biopsy
Open prostatic biopsy
Transurethral resection
Cytology of prostate secretions

Note: Carcinoma of the prostate may be detected as an incidental finding in the pathologic specimen obtained at transurethral resection for apparent benign prostatic hypertrophy.

Tumor Staging

Digital rectal examination
Excretory urography
Computerized tomography of pelvis to detect extension to seminal vesicles, bladder, and periprostatic soft tissues

LYMPH NODE COMPARTMENT

Lymph Node Signs and Symptoms

Lymph node involvement with prostatic carcinoma is usually asymptomatic.

Lymph Node Staging

Lymph node staging is particularly important if radical prostatectomy is planned.

Lymphography with percutaneous biopsy of suspicious lymphadenopathy, if clinically indicated
Computerized tomography
Surgical staging

Note: The need for lymph node staging is dependent on treatment philosophy. The choice of primary therapy with either surgery or irradiation remains controversial; therefore no standard staging recommendations can be offered.

METASTASIS COMPARTMENT

Metastasis Signs and Symptoms

Bone pain (Figure 3.59); bone is by far the most common metastatic site
Anemia

173

Weight loss

Fatigue

Azotemia due to obstructive uropathy

Supraclavicular or inguinal adenopathy

Dyspnea, cough due to lymphangitic pulmonary involvement

Evaluation for Metastasis

Plain films of painful bony sites

Isotope bone scan; a positive scan may precede radiographic changes by as much as 6 months

Chest x-ray films

Liver function tests

Liver imaging: if clinical suspicion of liver metastasis arises

Acid phosphatase, prostatic fraction: may be elevated in some cases of local disease and normal in some cases of metastatic disease; not highly reliable

TNM CLASSIFICATION OF PROSTATE CANCER

T: Primary Tumor

T0	No tumor palpable; includes incidental findings of cancer in a biopsy or operative specimen
T1	Intracapsular surrounded by normal gland
T2	Tumor confined to gland, deforming contour, and invading capsule, but lateral sulci and seminal vesicles are not involved
T3	Tumor extends beyond capsule with or without involvement of lateral sulci and/or seminal vesicles
T4	Tumor fixed or involving neighboring structures

N: Regional Lymph Nodes

N0	No involvement of regional lymph nodes
N1	Involvement of a single regional lymph node
N2	Involvement of multiple regional lymph nodes
N3	Free space between tumor and fixed pelvic wall mass
N4	Involvement of juxtaregional nodes

M: Distance Metastasis

MX Not assessed

M0 No (known) distant metastasis

M1 Distant metastasis present

Staging System for Prostate Cancer* (Figure 3.60)

Stage	A	Incidental finding
	A_1	Focal involvement
	A_2	Diffuse involvement
Stage	B	Confined to prostate
	B_1	Small discrete nodule
	B_2	Large or multiple nodules
Stage	C	Localized to periprostatic area
	C_1	No involvement of seminal vesicles
	C_2	Involvement of seminal vesicles
Stage	D	Metastatic disease
	D_1	Pelvic lymph node metastasis or ureteral obstruction causing hydronephrosis
	D_2	Bone or distant lymph node or organ or soft tissue metastasis

PATIENT EVALUATION DIAGRAM

See Figure 3.61.

* Reprinted with permission from Rosenthal SN, Bennett JM, eds: *Practical Cancer Chemotherapy.* Garden City, N.Y.: Medical Examination, 1981, p 274.

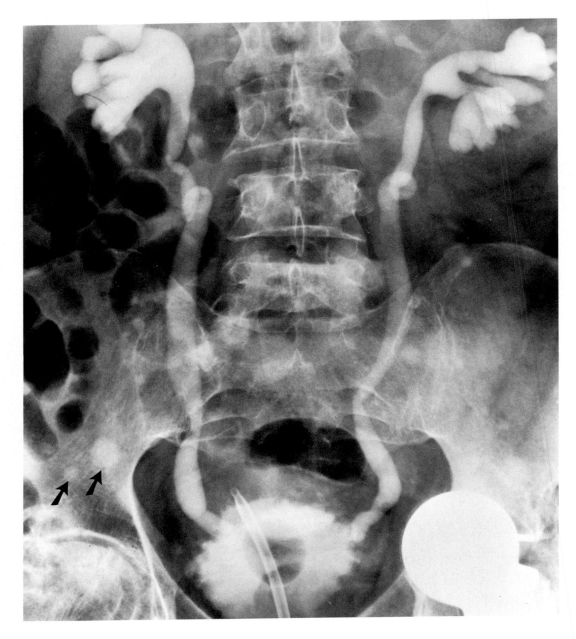

Figure 3.58 Bladder trabeculation and partial bilateral ureteral obstruction secondary to prostate enlargement (not directly visualized on this excretory urographic image). Note Foley catheter in the bladder as well as osteoblastic bone metastases (arrows). The presumptive diagnosis is metastatic carcinoma of the prostate.

176

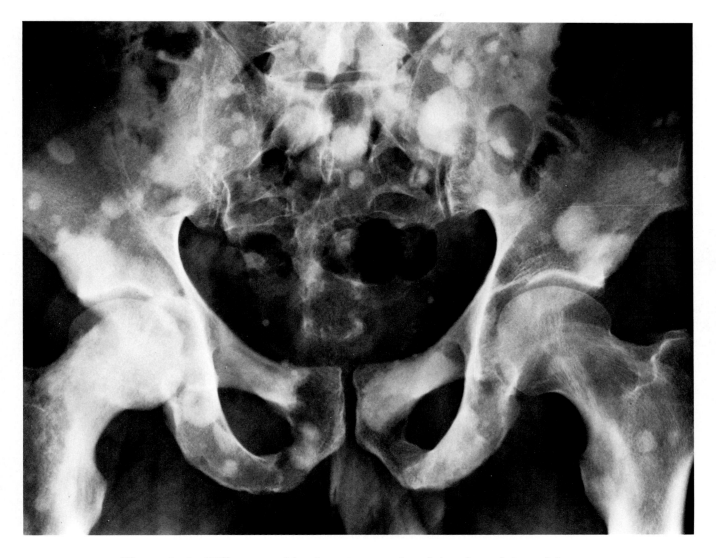

Figure 3.59 *Diffuse osteoblastic metastases involving the pelvis and femurs, typical of prostate carcinoma.*

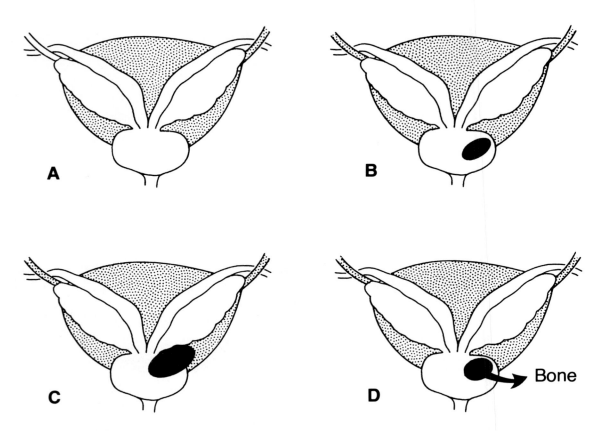

Figure 3.60 Staging classification of prostatic carcinoma.

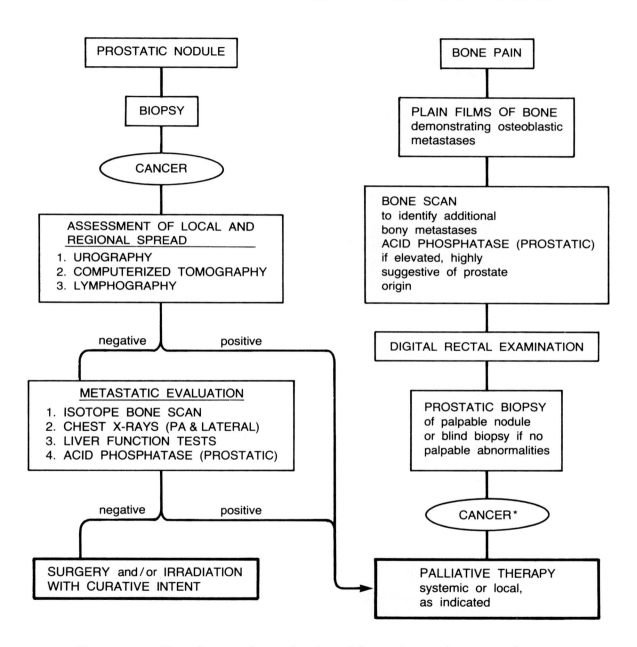

Figure 3.61 *Flow diagram for evaluation of the patient with suspected pros-*
*tate cancer. *Even in the face of a negative biopsy, a convincing clinical picture*
of metastatic prostate cancer warrants appropriate palliative therapy.

179

TESTICULAR CANCER

INCIDENCE

5,400 projected new cases in the U.S. in 1983
950 deaths
0.6% of new cancers in Americans and 1% of new cancers in American males
Most common cause of cancer deaths in 29- to 35-year-old males

EPIDEMIOLOGY

The etiology of testicular cancer is unknown, but the incidence is increased in cryptorchid and atrophic testes. Testicular cancer is rare in blacks, Africans, and Asians.

PATHOLOGY

Germ cell malignancies 90%
    Seminoma
    Nonseminomatous
        Embryonal
        Teratocarcinoma
        Choriocarcinoma
        Mixed
Nongerm cell malignancies 10%
    Lymphoma: most common testicular tumor in men over 60
    Interstitial cell tumor
    Gonadal-stromal tumors

TUMOR COMPARTMENT

Tumor Signs and Symptoms

Asymptomatic testicular mass
Mild testicular pain or tenderness

Tumor Diagnosis and Staging

Inguinal orchiectomy; trans-scrotal approach to be avoided
Beta human chorionic gonadotropin (β-HCG)

Alpha-fetoprotein (AFP); one or both markers (AFP and/or β-HCG) are elevated in the majority of patients with nonseminomatous germ cell cancers

LYMPH NODE COMPARTMENT

Lymph Node Signs and Symptoms

Usually asymptomatic

Back pain due to retroperitoneal adenopathy

Flank pain due to ureteral obstruction with hydronephrosis

Lymph Node Staging

Computerized tomography (Figure 3.62)

Lymphography (Figure 3.63); less reliable than CT since upper para-aortic and renal hilar nodes are not usually visualized with lymphography; CT is the preferred examination

Retroperitoneal lymphadenectomy for nonseminomatous germ cell tumors

METASTATIC COMPARTMENT

Metastasis Signs and Symptoms

Gynecomastia due to the effect of elevated HCG

Signs and symptoms of liver metastases

Dyspnea and chest pain

Supraclavicular adenopathy

Evaluation for Metastasis

Careful physical examination with particular attention to liver and lymph nodes

Chest x-ray films (Figure 3.64) to detect mediastinal adenopathy and pulmonary nodules

β-HCG and AFP assays

Liver function tests

Liver imaging; review liver images on CT performed for lymph node staging

Plain film or computerized whole lung tomography: only necessary in those cases with elevated serum markers and no clinical or radiologic evidence of metastatic disease

TNM CLASSIFICATION OF TESTICULAR CANCER

T: Primary Tumor

TX	Primary tumor assessment not carried out, or any category applicable
T0	No evidence of primary tumor
T1	Tumor limited to body of testis
T2	Tumor extending beyond tunica albuginea
T3	Tumor including rete testis or epididymis
T4a	Invasion of spermatic cord
T4b	Invasion of scrotal wall

N: Regional Lymph Nodes

NX	Regional lymph node assessment not carried out, or any category applicable
N0	No evidence of involved nodes
N1	Nodes not visibly enlarged at surgery but microscopic disease found on pathological exam
N1a	5 or fewer nodes +
N1b	>5 nodes +
N2	Nodes enlarged and microscopically contain tumor but not extension beyond nodes into areolar tissue
N2a	Largest node <2 cm and 5 or fewer nodes involved (both criteria)
N2b	Largest node >2 cm and/or more than 5 nodes involved
N3	Extension into adjacent areolar tissue (microscopic as well as gross); no gross residual tumor remaining after surgery
N4	Tumor present in retroperitoneal nodes, retroperitoneal areolar tissue with gross residual tumor remaining after surgery

M: Distant Metastases

MX	Complete assessment of distant metastases not carried out, or any category applicable
M0	No evidence of distant metastases
M1	Distant metastases present

STAGING SYSTEM FOR TESTICULAR CANCER

At least five overlapping, competing staging systems for testicular cancer are in current use, and no one system has yet achieved general acceptance. Therefore, to avoid confusion, a full tumor description using the TNM system should be listed for every patient.

PATIENT EVALUATION DIAGRAMS

See Figures 3.65 and 3.66.

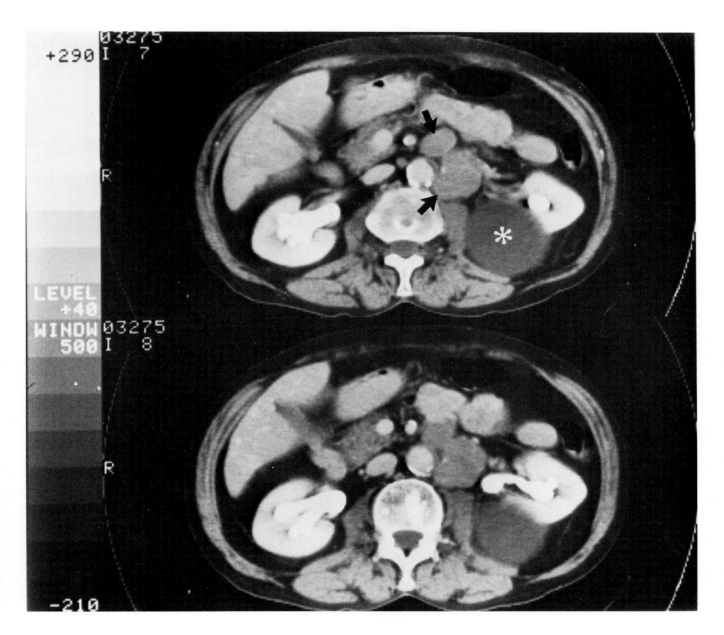

Figure 3.62 *Computerized tomogram showing left pararenal lymphadenop-athy (arrows). An incidental renal cyst is visualized (*).*

183

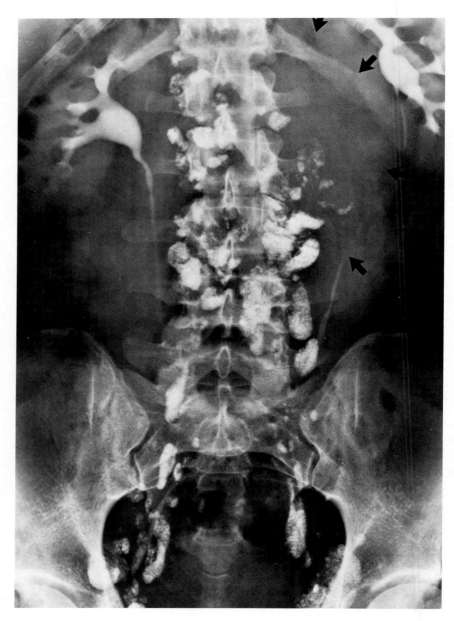

Figure 3.63 Single view from a lymphogram taken 24 hours after contrast injection. An excretory urogram was performed just prior to this film. Marked deformity of lymph nodes as well as a large mass medial to the left kidney (arrows) deviating the ureter laterally indicates lymph node involvement from a known left testicular cancer.

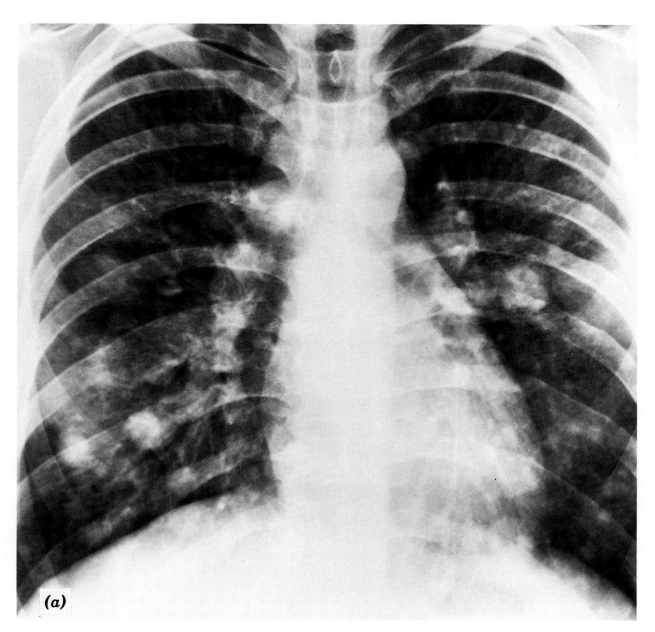

Figure 3.64 (a) Multiple pulmonary metastases are seen within both lungs in this patient with newly diagnosed testicular cancer.

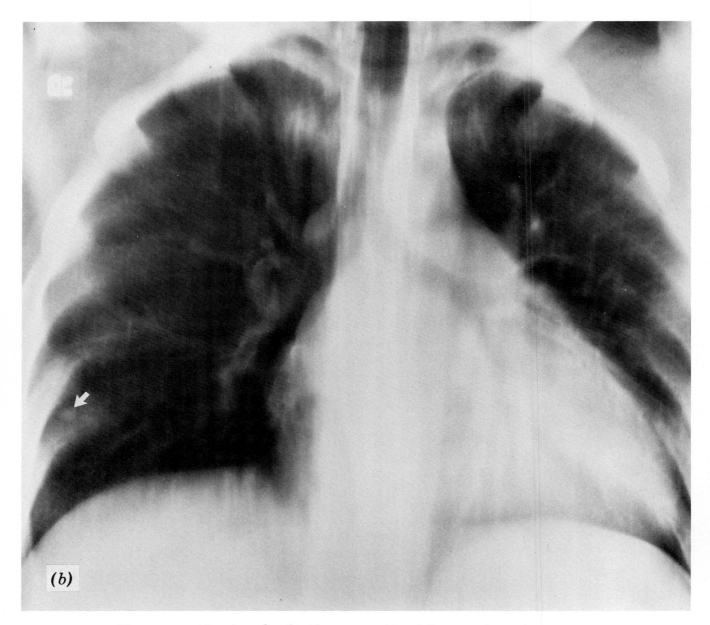

Figure 3.64 (Continued) *(b) Chest x-ray film following chemotherapy (not shown) was entirely clear, but whole lung tomograms revealed a single small right lower lobe nodule (arrow). This lesion was removed surgically and proved to be a fibrotic scar without any evidence of tumor. The patient remains free of disease 7 years after diagnosis.*

186

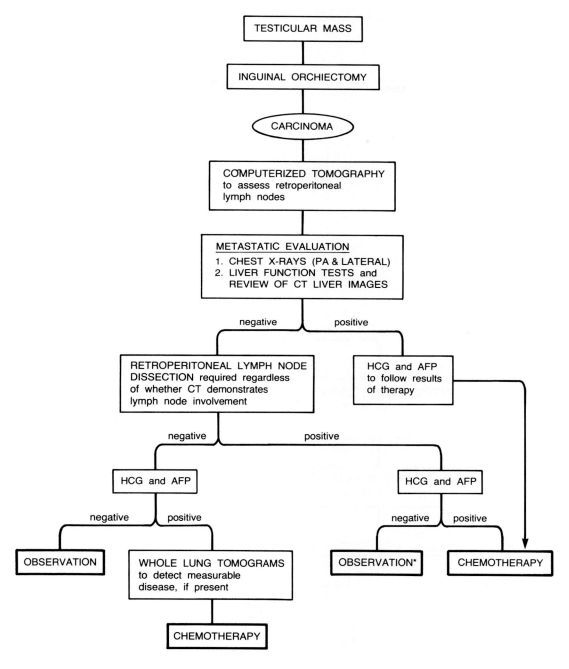

Figure 3.65 *Flow diagram for evaluation of the patient with suspected non-seminomatous germ cell carcinoma of the testis. * Retroperitoneal lymph node dissection is curative in some patients with involved lymph nodes.*

187

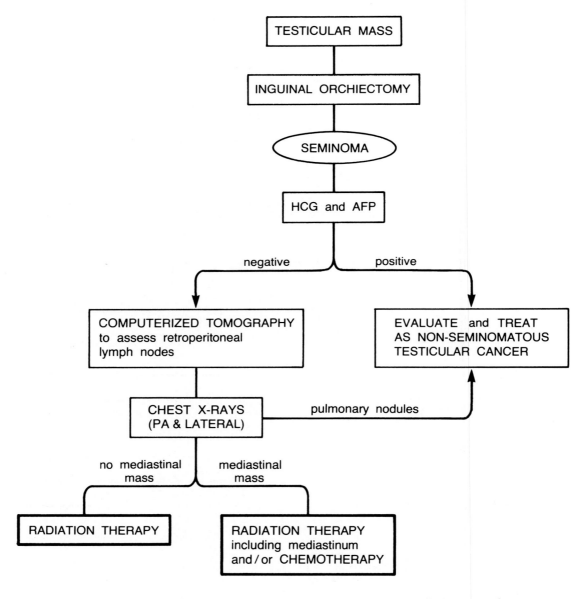

Figure 3.66 *Flow diagram for evaluation of the patient with suspected seminoma.*

OVARIAN CANCER

INCIDENCE

18,200 projected new cases in the U.S. in 1983
11,500 deaths
2.1% of new cancers in Americans and 4.3% of new cancers in American women

EPIDEMIOLOGY

An increased incidence of ovarian cancer is observed in industrialized countries, among women with breast cancer, nulliparous women, and in some families. The incidence of ovarian cancer is low in Asia and in developing countries.

PATHOLOGY

Eighty-five to 90% of ovarian cancers are adenocarcinomas; 10–15% are stromal and germ cell cancers. Ovarian adenocarcinomas spread almost exclusively by peritoneal dissemination and contiguous extension. Therefore, the concept of lymph node and metastasis compartments has less relevance to the evaluation of patients with this disease.

SIGNS AND SYMPTOMS

Early stage ovarian cancer is usually asymptomatic; a majority of patients have advanced disease at the time of initial presentation. Most signs and symptoms are related to advanced disease.

Abdominal and pelvic pain
Increased abdominal girth due to tumor bulk and/or ascites
Nausea, early satiety, weight loss
Dysfunctional or postmenopausal bleeding
Dyspnea due to ascites or pleural effusion
Abdominal or pelvic mass

PRESURGICAL STAGING

Thorough pelvic examination
Chest x-ray films (Figure 3.67)

Paracentesis and thoracentesis if effusions are present

Pelvic ultrasonography or computerized tomography (Figure 3.68) if pelvic examination is equivocal

Lymphography reliably detects para-aortic adenopathy, but proper surgical staging usually makes lymphography unnecessary

SURGICAL STAGING

Inspection and palpation of both ovaries and other pelvic structures

Inspection, palpation, and biopsy of omentum, undersurfaces of diaphragms, liver, peritoneal surfaces, para-aortic lymph nodes

Peritoneal washings

Biopsies of any suspicious areas

FIGO STAGING SYSTEM FOR OVARIAN CANCER

Stage I	Growth limited to the ovaries
Stage Ia	Growth limited to one ovary; no ascites
	1. No tumor on the external surface; capsule intact
	2. Tumor present on the external surface or capsule ruptured
Stage Ib	Growth limited to both ovaries; no ascites
	1. No tumor on the external surface; capsules intact
	2. Tumor present on the external surface or capsules ruptured
Stage Ic	Tumor either stage Ia or stage Ib but with ascites or positive peritoneal washings
Stage II	Growth involving one or both ovaries with pelvic extension
Stage IIa	Extension or metastases to the uterus or tubes
Stage IIb	Extension to other pelvic tissues
Stage IIc	Tumor either stage IIa or stage IIb, but with ascites present or positive washings
Stage III	Growth involving one or both ovaries with intraperitoneal metastases outside the pelvis or positive retroperitoneal nodes; tumor limited to the true pelvis with histologically proven malignant extension to the omentum or small bowel
Stage IV	Growth involving one or both ovaries with distant metastases; if pleural effusion is present, there must be positive cytology to allot a case to stage IV; parenchymal liver metastases equal stage IV

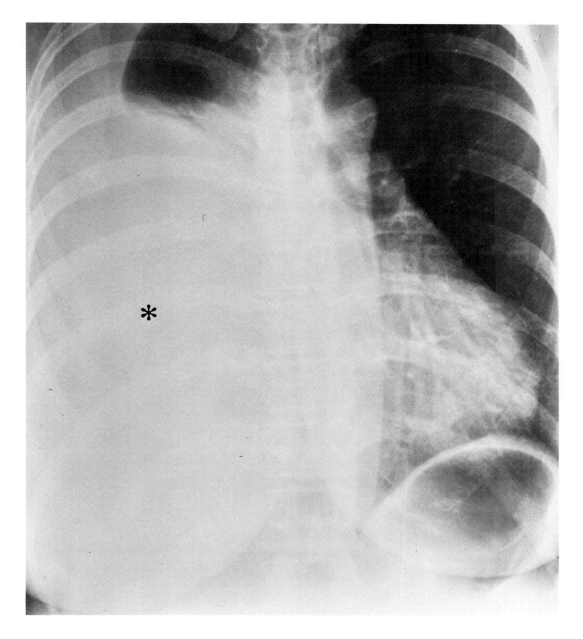

Figure 3.67 Large right pleural effusion (*) in a woman presenting with ascites and a pelvis mass—a common triad in ovarian carcinoma.

191

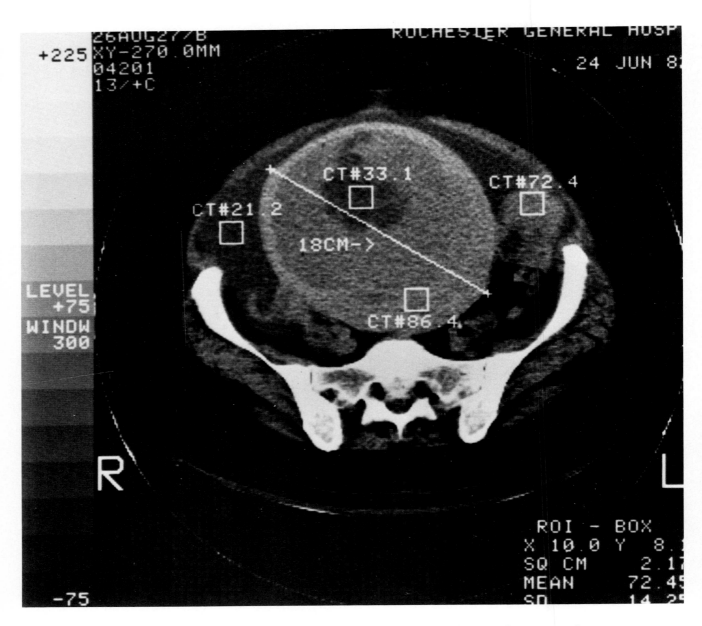

Figure 3.68 *Computerized tomogram of the pelvis showing a large complex mass which proved to be an ovarian carcinoma.*

ENDOMETRIAL CANCER

INCIDENCE

39,000 projected new cases in the U.S. in 1983

3,000 deaths

4.7% of new cancers in Americans and 9.2% of new cancers in American women

Most comon gynecologic malignancy

Incidence has been increasing rapidly in recent years

EPIDEMIOLOGY

Risk factors for endometrial carcinoma include obesity, hypertension, nulliparity, and diabetes. The disease is more common among Jewish women. Excessive estrogen levels, both endogenous and exogenous, appear to cause endometrial carcinoma, and the incidence is increased among women who take estrogens for menopausal symptoms and among those with Stein-Leventhal syndrome, granulosa-theca tumors of the ovary, and anovulatory menstrual cycles, all of which are associated with increased estrogen levels. The incidence of endometrial carcinoma is also higher in industrialized western countries than it is in Asia.

PATHOLOGY

Over 90% are adenocarcinomas; some have squamous elements and are termed adenocanthomas or adenosquamous carcinomas. The remainder are mesenchymal tumors—mixed müllerian tumors and endometrial sarcomas.

TUMOR COMPARTMENT

Tumor Signs and Symptoms

Postmenopausal bleeding

Abnormal menstrual pattern in premenopausal women

Tissue Diagnosis

Pap smear (with endocervical and vaginal pool cytologies)

Endometrial biopsy

Tumor Staging

Pelvic examination under anesthesia (EUA)

Rectal examination

Fractional curettage

Multiple cervical biopsies

Urography for localization of ureters before major pelvic surgery and for kidney localization before irradiation

Cystoscopy or computerized tomography if bladder involvement suspected

Barium enema, computerized tomography (Figure 3.69), or proctosigmoidoscopy if colorectal involvement suspected

LYMPH NODE COMPARTMENT

Lymph Node Signs and Symptoms

Back pain due to para-aortic lymph node metastasis or ureteral obstruction

Lymph Node Staging

Para-aortic lymph node involvement is assessed with lymphography and percutaneous lymph node biopsy in patients with stage II or stage III disease. Most patients with stage I disease do not require lymphography, since their risk of para-aortic lymph node involvement is low; however, stage I patients with poorly differentiated cancers (G3) are at greater risk and should undergo preoperative lymphography.

METASTASIS COMPARTMENT

Distant dissemination of disease is unusual at the time of diagnosis. Routine metastatic evaluation, other than chest x-ray films, is unwarranted in the absence of clinical indication of metastatic disease.

FIGO STAGING SYSTEM

Stage 0	Carcinoma in situ; histological findings suspicious of malignancy
Stage I	The carcinoma is confined to the corpus including the isthmus
Stage Ia	The length of the uterine cavity is 8 cm or less
Stage Ib	The length of the uterine cavity is more than 8 cm

The stage I case should be subgrouped with regard to the histologic type of the adenocarcinoma as follows:

G1	Highly differentiated adenomatous carcinoma
G2	Differentiated adenomatous carcinoma with partly solid areas
G3	Predominantly solid or entirely undifferentiated carcinoma
Stage II	The carcinoma has involved the corpus and the cervix but has not extended outside the uterus
Stage III	The carcinoma has extended outside the uterus but not outside the true pelvis
Stage IV	The carcinoma has extended outside the true pelvis or has obviously involved the mucosa of the bladder or rectum; bullous edema as such does not permit a case to be allotted to stage IV
Stage IVa	Spread of the growth to adjacent organs
Stage IVb	Spread to distant organs

PATIENT EVALUATION DIAGRAM

See Figure 3.70.

195

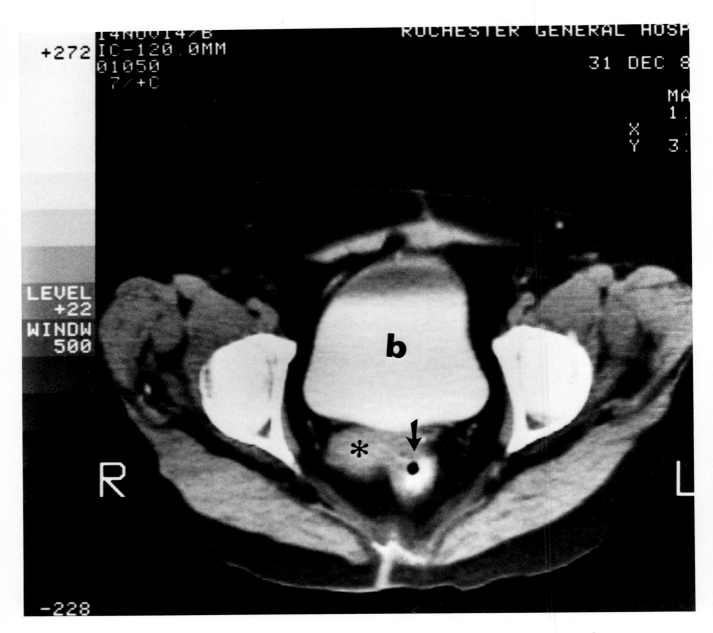

Figure 3.69 *Computerized tomogram of the pelvis in which an endometrial cancer (*) is seen invading the rectum (arrow) behind the contrast-filled bladder (b).*

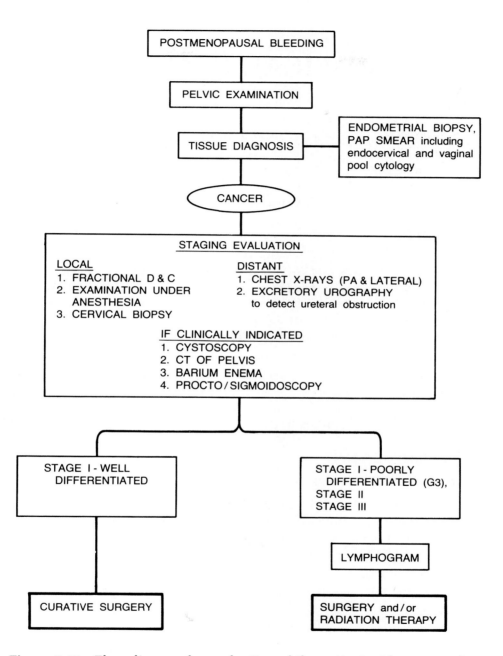

Figure 3.70 *Flow diagram for evaluation of the patient with suspected endometrial carcinoma.*

CERVICAL CANCER

INCIDENCE

16,000 projected new cases in the U.S. in 1983

7,000 deaths

1.9% of new cancers in Americans and 3.8% of new cancers in American women

Incidence decreasing steadily in U.S.

EPIDEMIOLOGY

Increased risk of cervical carcinoma is seen among Puerto Rican and black women, women of lower socioeconomic status, those with early sexual activity, multiple sexual partners, and early age at first pregnancy. The incidence is lower among Jewish women and Fiji Islanders, nulliparous women, and nuns. A relationship with genital herpes infection appears to exist. In utero exposure to diethylstilbestrol leads to an increased incidence of clear cell carcinoma of the vagina and cervix.

PATHOLOGY

Over 90% are squamous cell carcinomas, while the remainder are adenocarcinomas and clear cell carcinomas.

TUMOR COMPARTMENT

Tumor Signs and Symptoms

Most cases of in situ and early invasive cervical carcinomas are asymptomatic and are detected by routine cytologic screening. Patients with advanced cervical carcinoma frequently have a long history of chronic cervicitis, severe dysplasia, and carcinoma in situ. Symptoms include

Postcoital spotting

Metrorrhagia (intermenstrual bleeding)

Menorrhagia

Serosanguinous vaginal discharge

Pelvic pain

Urinary and rectal symptoms in advanced stages (hematuria, urinary urgency, rectal pain, bleeding, tenesmus)

TUMOR STAGING

Pelvic and rectal examination

Pap smear

Schiller test with directed cervical biopsies

Colposcopy

Conization

Multiple punch biopsies of cervix

Examination under anesthesia

Cystoscopy, proctosigmoidoscopy, barium enema, except for stage 0 and stage Ia

Excretory urography

LYMPH NODE COMPARTMENT

Lymph Node Signs and Symptoms

Back pain due to para-aortic lymph node involvement

Azotemia due to obstructive uropathy

Lymphedema of one or both legs

Lymph Node Diagnosis and Staging

Computerized tomography (Figure 3.71); detects bulky lymph node involvement

Lymphography (Figure 3.72); more sensitive than CT

Percutaneous biopsy of suspicious lymph nodes under lymphographic or CT guidance

Note: Lymph node staging is omitted in stage 0 and stage Ia disease.

METASTASIS COMPARTMENT

Distant dissemination of disease is unusual at the time of diagnosis. Routine metastatic evaluation, other than careful physical examination and chest x-ray films, is unnecessary in the absence of clinical indications.

FIGO STAGING SYSTEM FOR CERVICAL CANCER

Preinvasive Carcinoma

Stage 0   Carcinoma in situ, intraepithelial carcinoma

Invasive Carcinoma

Stage I	Carcinoma strictly confined to the cervix (extension to the corpus should be disregarded)
Stage Ia	Microinvasive carcinoma (early stromal invasion)
Stage Ib	All other cases of stage I; occult cancer should be marked "occ"
Stage II	The carcinoma extends beyond the cervix, but has not extended onto the pelvic wall; the carcinoma involves the vagina, but not the lower third
Stage IIa	No obvious parametrial involvement
Stage IIb	Obvious parametrial involvement
Stage III	The carcinoma has extended onto the pelvic wall; on rectal examination there is no cancer-free space between the tumor and the pelvic wall; the tumor involves the lower third of the vagina; all cases with a hydronephrosis or nonfunctioning kidney
Stage IIIa	No extension onto the pelvic wall
Stage IIIb	Extension onto the pelvic wall and/or hydronephrosis or nonfunctioning kidney
Stage IV	The carcinoma has extended beyond the true pelvis or has clinically involved the mucosa of the bladder or rectum; bullous edema as such does not permit a case to be allotted to stage IV
Stage IVa	Spread of the growth to adjacent organs
Stage IVb	Spread to distant organs

PATIENT EVALUATION DIAGRAM

See Figure 3.73.

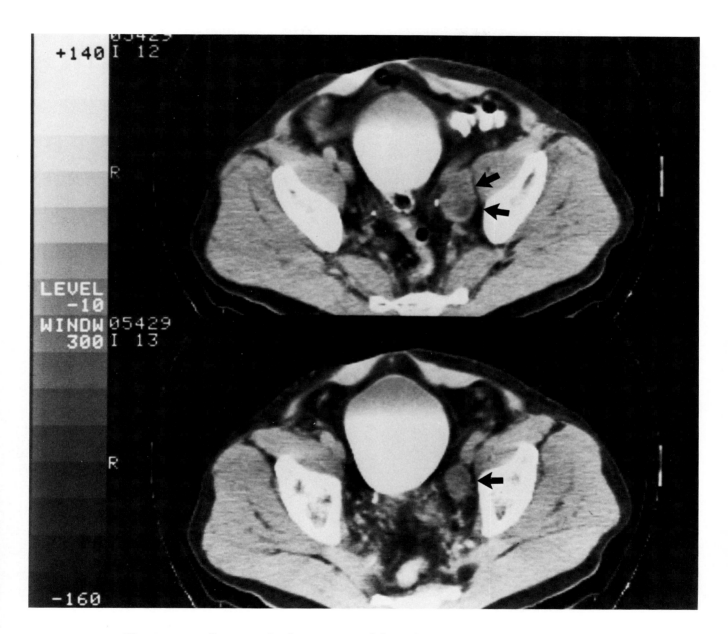

Figure 3.71 Computerized tomogram of the pelvis demonstrating pelvic side-wall lymphadenopathy (arrows) in a patient with carcinoma of the cervix.

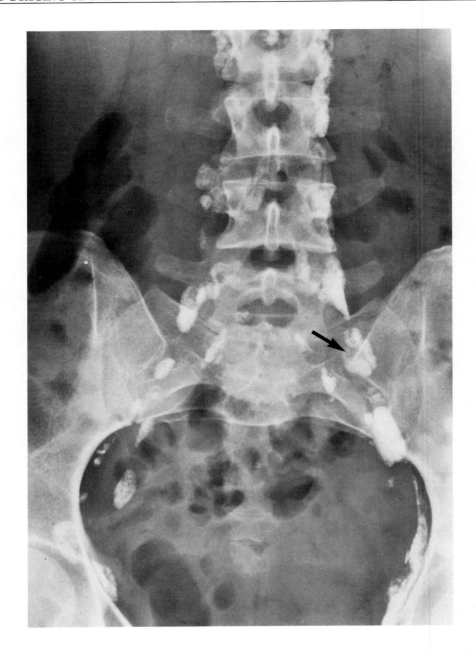

Figure 3.72 Lymphogram showing a small filling defect (arrow) in a left iliac lymph node. Percutaneous biopsy of this lesion confirmed the diagnosis of cervical carcinoma. (Courtesy of Dr. Francis Burgener)

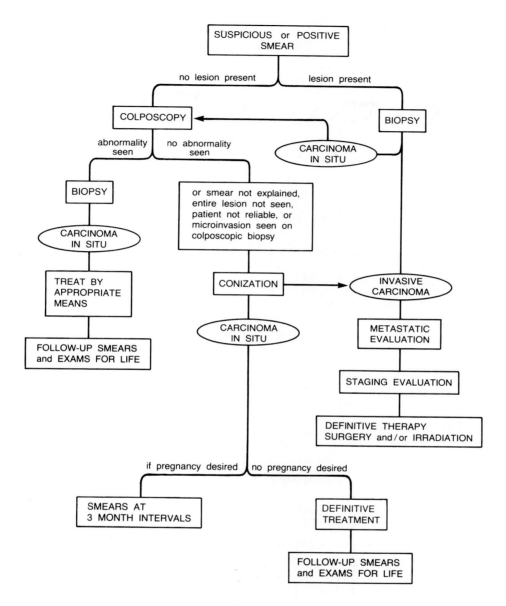

Figure 3.73 *Flow diagram for evaluation of the patient with an abnormal cervical smear. Detailed assessment for lymph node and metastatic involvement depends on the apparent stage as determined at the time of biopsy and examination under anesthesia. The full staging evaluation should be performed under the joint direction of the gynecologic surgeon and radiation oncologist. (Adapted with permission from Nelson JH, Averett HE, Richart RM: Detection, diagnostic evaluation and treatment of dysplasia and early carcinoma of the cervix. CA **25:**138, 1975.)*

MALIGNANT MELANOMA

INCIDENCE

17,400 projected new cases in the U.S. in 1983
5,200 deaths
2% of new cancers in Americans
Male:female ratio 1.0
Incidence is increasing rapidly, with a doubling every 10–17 years

EPIDEMIOLOGY

The risk of melanoma is high in fair-skinned, freckled patients who sunburn easily; the risk is low in blacks and Asians. An etiologic relationship to sunlight is clear; in every geographic area studied the incidence of melanoma rises as the latitude approaches 0° (equator). In some families melanoma is hereditary.

TUMOR COMPARTMENT

Tumor Signs and Symptoms

Pigmented skin lesion with:

Variegated color   Increase in size
Irregular surface   Ulceration
Bleeding   Change in color
Itching

Tumor Diagnosis and Staging

Excisional or incisional biopsy, depending on lesion size
Staging is surgical-pathological

LYMPH NODE COMPARTMENT

Lymph Node Signs and Symptoms

Local or regional lymphadenopathy
Lymphedema of an extremity

Lymph Node Staging

Physical examination
Surgical staging (in some cases)

METASTASIS COMPARTMENT

Routine chest x-ray films are recommended at the time of diagnosis to detect occult pulmonary metastases. Because of the low positive yield of additional metastatic evaluations in asymptomatic patients at initial presentation, routine bone, brain, and liver imaging is not warranted. Specific imaging should be performed based on clinical concern (Figure 3.74).

Malignant melanoma may metastasize to any organ or site with protean manifestations. Symptoms not usually associated with metastatic disease, such as upper gastrointestinal bleeding or hematuria, should raise suspicion of metastasis in patients with melanoma.

CLARK'S LEVELS OF INVASION OF PRIMARY MALIGNANT MELANOMA (Figure 3.75)

Level I: Melanoma limited to the epidermis (above the basal lamina); this is actually in situ disease and quite rare

Level II: Melanoma extends through the basement membrane into the papillary dermis

Level III: Melanoma fills and widens the papillary dermis at the interface with the reticular dermis

Level IV: Melanoma penetrates into the reticular dermis

Level V: Melanoma extends into the subcutaneous tissue

An alternative to the Clark classification is to measure the actual depth or thickness of the primary lesion with an optical micrometer. Both systems correlate closely with prognosis.

A TNM system for malignant melanoma exists but is not widely used.

CLINICAL STAGING SYSTEM FOR MALIGNANT MELANOMA

Stage I   Localized primary melanoma or locally recurrent melanoma following previous excision

Stage II   Primary melanoma with metastases limited to regional lymph nodes; in most cases stage II represents patients with palpable regional adenopathy, since elective lymphadenectomies in patients with clinically uninvolved lymph nodes are no longer routinely performed

Stage III   Widespread disease

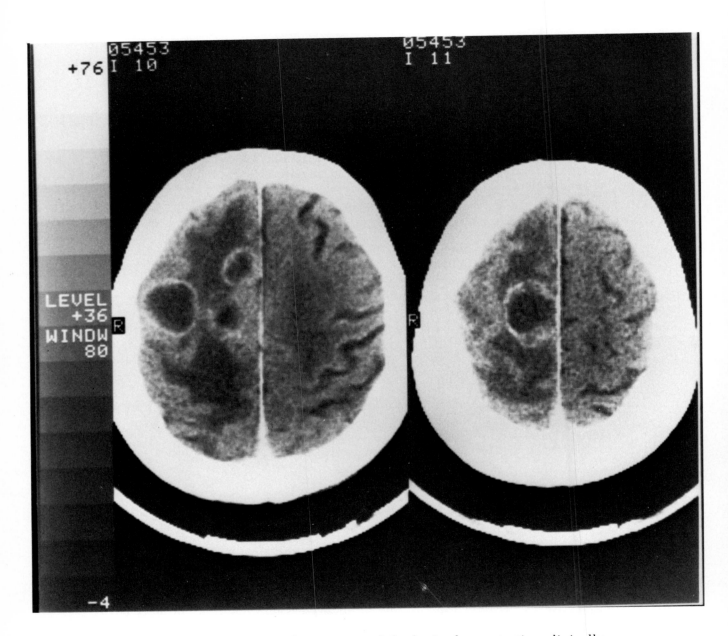

Figure 3.74 Computerized tomogram of the brain demonstrating clinically suspected metastases in a patient with malignant melanoma.

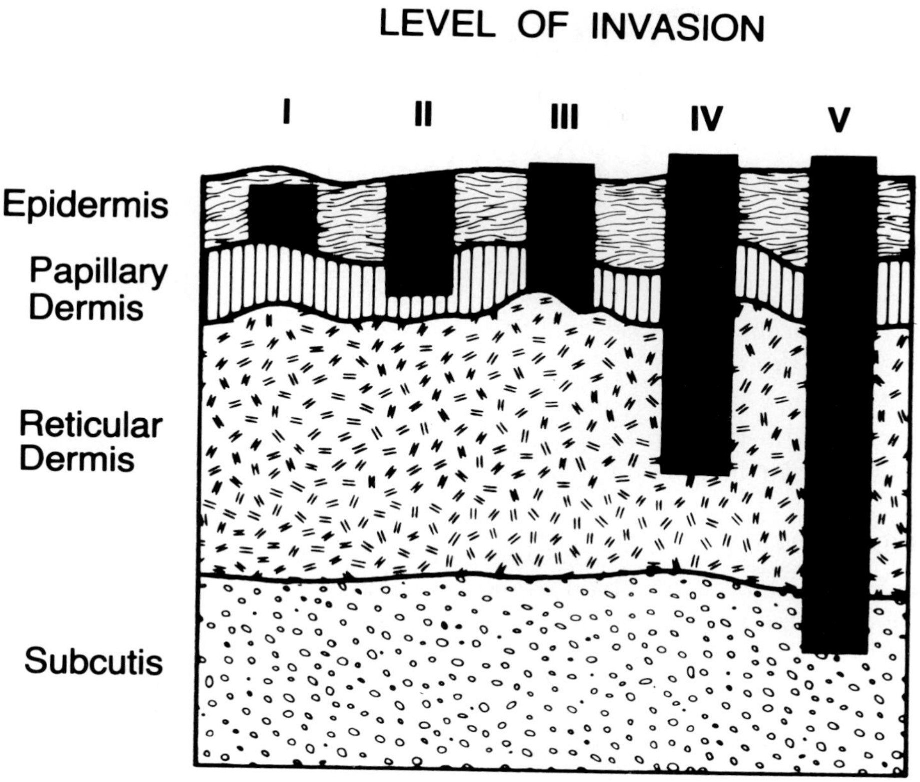

LEVEL OF INVASION

Figure 3.75 *Clark's levels of invasion of malignant melanoma.*

HODGKIN'S AND NON-HODGKIN'S LYMPHOMAS

INCIDENCE

Hodgkin's Disease
7,100 projected new cases in 1983
1,600 deaths
0.8% of new cancers
Male:female ratio 1.3
Bimodal age distribution

Non-Hodgkin's Lymphoma
23,600 projected new cases in 1983
12,300 deaths
2.8% of new cancers
Male:female ratio 1.0
Incidence rises with age

EPIDEMIOLOGY

Increased risk of developing lymphoma is associated with the following conditions: primary and acquired immunodeficiency states, chronic immunosuppressive therapy, Sjögren's syndrome, rheumatoid arthritis, systemic lupus erythematosus, Klinefelter's syndrome, exposure to ionizing radiation, and long-term hydantoin therapy. Evidence for an association of the Epstein-Barr virus with Burkitt's lymphoma is strong, but a causative relationship has not been proved.

PATHOLOGY

Hodgkin's disease
    Lymphocyte predominant
    Nodular sclerosis
    Mixed cellularity
    Lymphocyte depletion

Non-Hodgkin's lymphomas: modified Rappaport classification

Favorable Histologies (Figure 3.76)
Nodular poorly differentiated lymphocytic (NPDL)
Nodular mixed lymphocytic-histiocytic (NM)
Diffuse well-differentiated lymphocytic (DWDL)

Unfavorable Histologies (Figure 3.77)
Diffuse poorly differentiated lymphocytic (DPDL)
Diffuse mixed lymphocytic-histiocytic (DM)
Diffuse histiocytic (DH)
Diffuse undifferentiated (DU)
Lymphoblastic (LB)
Nodular histiocytic (NH)

	Favorable	*Unfavorable*
Natural History:	Long, indolent course Multiple recurrences	Aggressive, rapidly fatal course unless treated to complete response
Treatment:	Nonintensive, palliative treatment	Intensive, curative treatment

CLINICAL MANIFESTATIONS

Painless adenopathy, either single or multiple
Hepatosplenomegaly
Mediastinal mass, superior vena cava syndrome
Ureteral obstruction
Spinal cord compression
Tracheal or bronchial compression
Venous obstruction of an extremity
Lytic or blastic bone lesions
Gastrointestinal tract lesions
Bone marrow failure
Pulmonary parenchymal lesions
Pleural effusions
Skin nodules
Systemic symptoms: fever, weight loss, night sweats, pruritus

TISSUE DIAGNOSIS

Tissue is usually obtained by surgical biopsy of an enlarged lymph node. On occasion laparotomy, endoscopy, mediastinal exploration, bone biopsy, or other procedures are required in patients who do not present with readily accessible peripheral lymphadenopathy. Lymph node tissue, however, is preferable, since pathologic subclassification of the lymphomas depends on their morphology in involved nodes.

STAGING EVALUATION

Careful physical examination with special attention to lymph node-bearing areas

Complete blood count and differential

Screening blood chemistries (including tests of liver and renal function)

Chest x-ray films (Figure 3.78)

Retroperitoneal lymph node imaging:

Computerized tomography (Figure 3.79) yields the most information and can assess mesenteric and porta hepatis nodes as well as retroperitoneal and pelvic nodes

Lymphography (Figure 3.80) demonstrates lymphomatous involvement with greater specificity than CT, but does not visualize upper para-aortic and mesenteric nodes that are readily imaged with CT

Ultrasonography (Figure 3.81) is less useful than CT for complete abdominal lymph node assessment; however, the low cost of ultrasonography makes it an attractive modality for serial evaluation of a previously detected abnormality

Bone marrow aspiration and biopsy for certain histologies and stages

Additional studies if clinically indicated:

Computerized tomography of the chest to detect pulmonary invasion in patients with mediastinal involvement

Thoracentesis, paracentesis if effusions present

Spinal tap with cerebrospinal fluid cytology for certain histologies and stages

Bone scan and plain films of involved areas

Barium studies of the gastrointestinal tract for patients presenting with gastrointestinal symptoms

Gallium scan; rarely useful

Staging laparotomy; primarily for Hodgkin's disease

STAGING SYSTEM (Ann Arbor Classification)

Stage I	Involvement of a single lymph node region (I) or a single extralymphatic organ or site (I_E)
Stage II	Involvement of two or more lymph node regions on the same side of the diaphragm (II) or localized involvement of an extralymphatic organ or site and of one or more lymph node regions on the same side of the diaphragm (II_E)
Stage III	Involvement of lymph node regions on both sides of the diaphragm (III) or localized involvement of an extralymphatic organ or site (III_E) or spleen (III_S) or both (III_{SE})
Stage IV	Diffuse or disseminated involvement of one or more extralymphatic organs with or without associated lymph node involvement

All stages   A = asymptomatic
                      B = fever, sweats, weight loss >10% of body weight

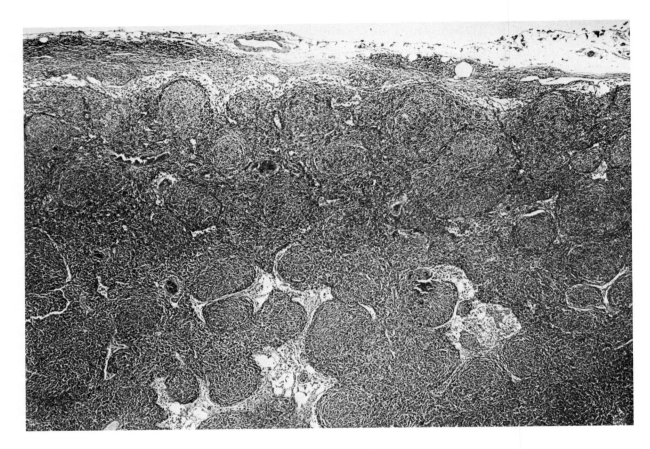

Figure 3.76 Low power photomicrograph of a lymph node containing a nodular lymphoma.

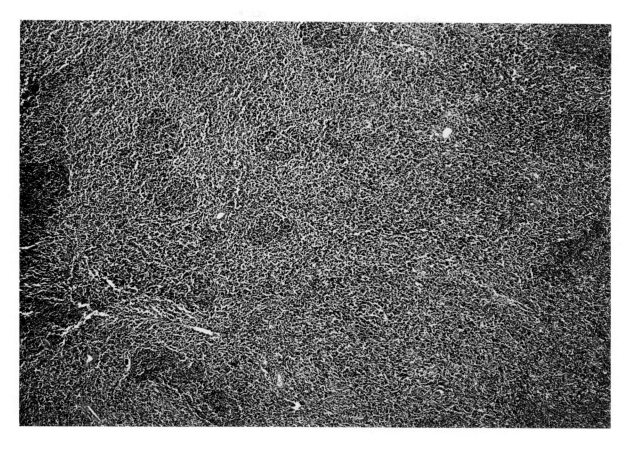

Figure 3.77 *Low power photomicrograph of a lymph node containing a diffuse lymphoma.*

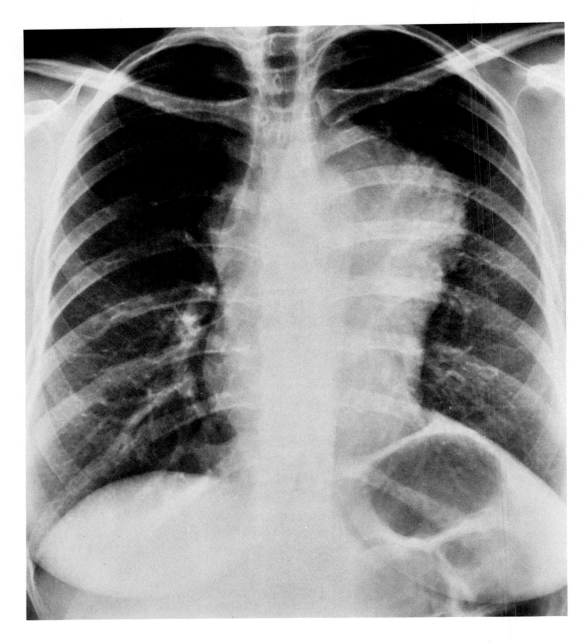

Figure 3.78 *Large left mediastinal mass in a patient with nodular sclerosing Hodgkin's disease.*

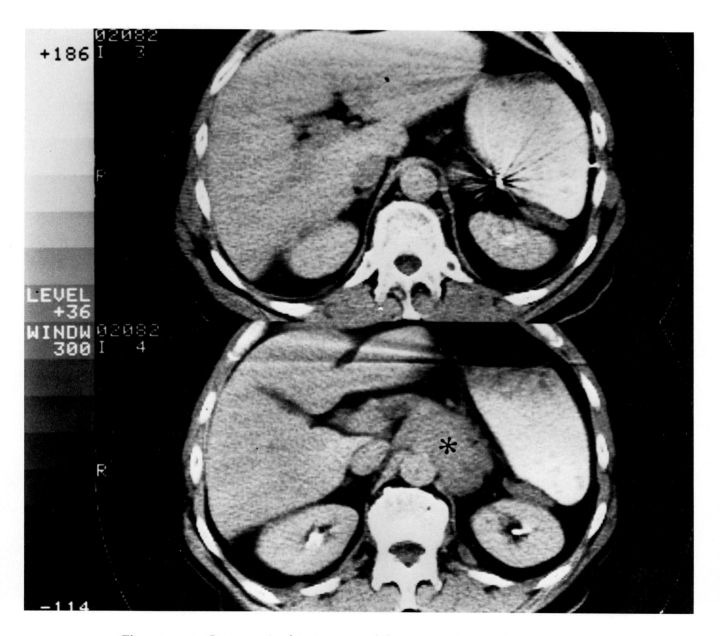

Figure 3.79 Computerized tomogram of the upper abdomen demonstrating left para-aortic adenopathy (*) in a patient who presented with cervical and mediastinal Hodgkin's disease.

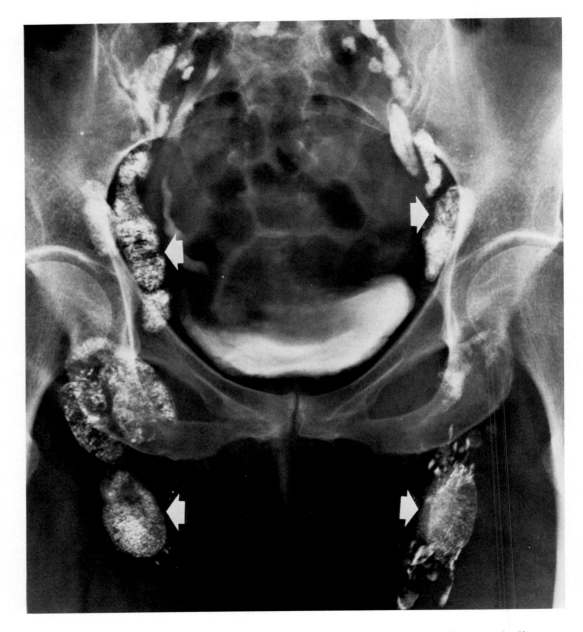

Figure 3.80 Lymphographic image with excretory urogram showing bulky lymph nodes (arrows) in the inguinal and iliac regions in a patient with non-Hodgkin's lymphoma.

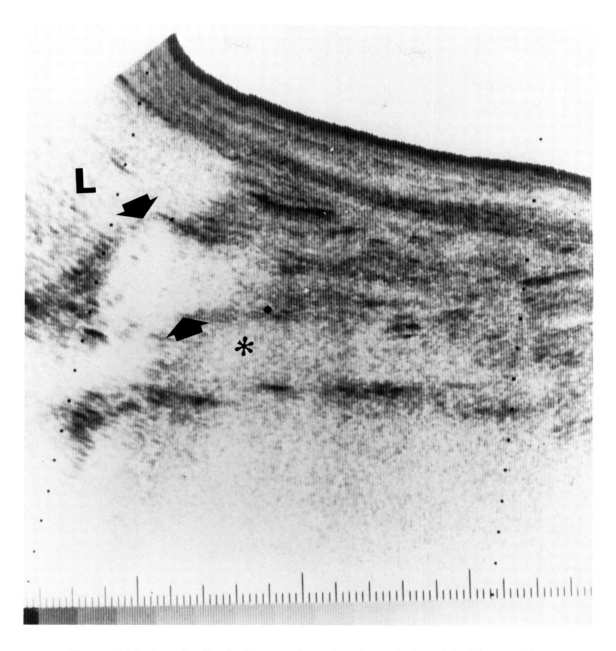

Figure 3.81 *Longitudinal ultrasound section through the mid-abdomen. En-*
larged lymph nodes (arrows) are seen just anterior to the aorta (*). L, liver.

SARCOMAS

INCIDENCE

Soft Tissue Sarcomas
4,800 projected new cases in U.S. in 1983
1,650 deaths
0.6% of new cancers but 6.5% of cancers in children under 15
Male:female ratio 1.2

Bone Sarcomas
1,900 projected new cases

1,750 deaths
0.2% of new cancers but 4.6% of cancers in children under 15
Male:female ratio 1.4

EPIDEMIOLOGY

The etiology of the sarcomas is unknown, but an increased incidence of certain sarcomas is seen in patients with various benign conditions, including basal cell nevus syndrome, neurofibromatosis, tuberous sclerosis, Werner's syndrome, intestinal polyposis, Paget's disease of bone, and chronic lymphedema following radical mastectomy. Kaposi's sarcoma, common in equatorial Africa, has recently occurred in epidemic form among male homosexuals and others with acquired immunodeficiency syndrome, AIDS.

PATHOLOGY

Tissue of Origin	Malignant Tumor	Usual Site	Comment
Fibrous	Fibrosarcoma	Lower limbs, trunk	Common
Adipose	Liposarcoma	Lower limbs, retroperitoneum	Common
Striated muscle	Rhabdomyosarcoma	Popliteal, gluteal, interscapular, orbit	Most common type in children
Smooth muscle	Leiomyosarcoma		
Synovial	Synovial sarcoma	Knee, ankle	
Nerve	Neurofibrosarcoma		Neurofibromatosis
Vascular	Angiosarcoma, lymphangiosarcoma, malignant hemangiopericytoma, Kaposi's sarcoma		

Tissue of Origin	Malignant Tumor	Usual Site	Comment
Histiocyte	Malignant fibrous histiocytoma, giant cell sarcoma		
Mesothelial	Malignant mesothelioma	Pleura	Asbestos exposure
Bone	Osteosarcoma	Knee	Paget's disease of bone
Bone	Chondrosarcoma	Pelvis, femur	
Bone	Ewing's sarcoma		Children and young adults

SOFT TISSUE SARCOMAS

Tumor Signs and Symptoms

Asymptomatic soft tissue mass

Symptoms due to tumor compression of adjacent structures

Tumor Diagnosis and Staging

Computerized tomography (Figure 3.82) for demonstration of anatomic extent and local invasion of adjacent structures, i.e., bone

Surgical biopsy

Angiography for vascular mapping if required for presurgical planning

Evaluation for Metastasis

Plain film or computerized tomography of the lungs*

Liver imaging for patients with retroperitoneal sarcomas

BONE SARCOMAS

Tumor Signs and Symptoms

Pain

Swelling and tenderness

Pathologic fracture

* Note: The lung is almost invariably the first site of metastatic involvement in patients with most soft tissue and bone sarcomas, and detailed assessment of the lungs is critical in patients who are candidates for radical surgery.

Tumor Diagnosis and Staging

Plain radiograph of involved bone (Figure 3.83)

Radiographic bone survey or bone scan to detect multifocal primary tumors, i.e., Ewing's and osteogenic sarcoma

Serum alkaline phosphatase

Percutaneous or surgical biopsy

Evaluation for Metastasis

Plain film or computerized tomography of the lungs*

TNM CLASSIFICATION FOR SOFT TISSUE SARCOMAS

T: Primary Tumor

T1   Tumor 5 cm or less in diameter
T2   Tumor more than 5 cm in diameter
T3   Tumor that grossly involves bone, major vessel, or major nerve

N: Regional Lymph Nodes

N0   No histologically verified metastases to lymph nodes
N1   Histologically verified regional lymph node metastasis

M: Distant Metastasis

M0   No distant metastasis
M1   Distant metastasis present

G: Histologic Grade

G1   Well differentiated
G2   Moderately well differentiated
G3   Poorly differentiated

STAGING SYSTEM FOR SOFT TISSUE SARCOMAS

Stage I:
    Stage IA   G1 T1 N0 M0
    Stage IB   G1 T2 N0 M0
Stage II:
    Stage IIA   G2 T1 N0 M0
    Stage IIB   G2 T2 N0 M0
Stage III:
    Stage IIIA   G3 T1 N0 M0
    Stage IIIB   G3 T2 N0 M0
Stage IV:
    Stage IVA   Any G T3 N0–1 M0
    Stage IVB   Any M1

No TNM or other staging system is available for sarcomas of bone.

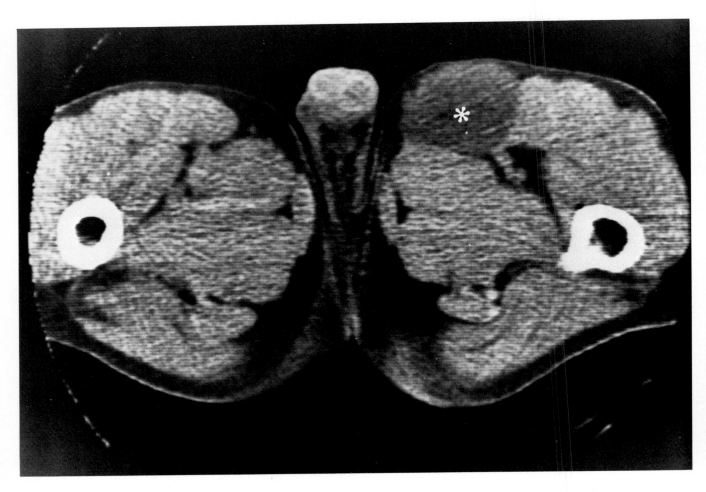

Figure 3.82 *Soft tissue sarcoma (*) seen within the anterior compartment of the left thigh. The opposite normal thigh is present, for comparison.*

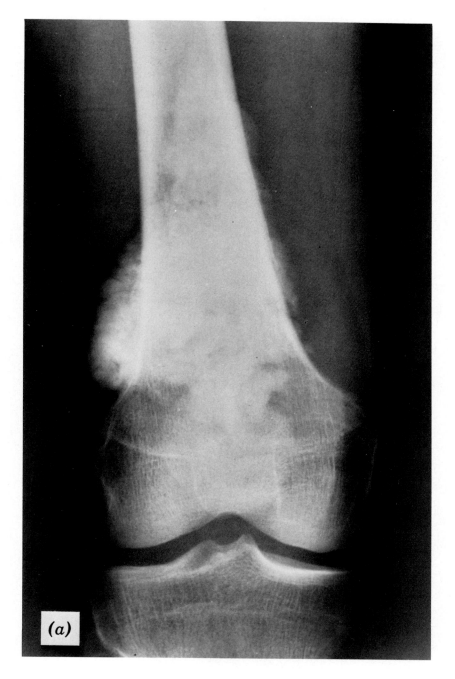

Figure 3.83 (a,b) Radiographic appearance of osteogenic sarcoma involving the distal femur. Note the exuberant periosteal new bone deposition posteriorly.

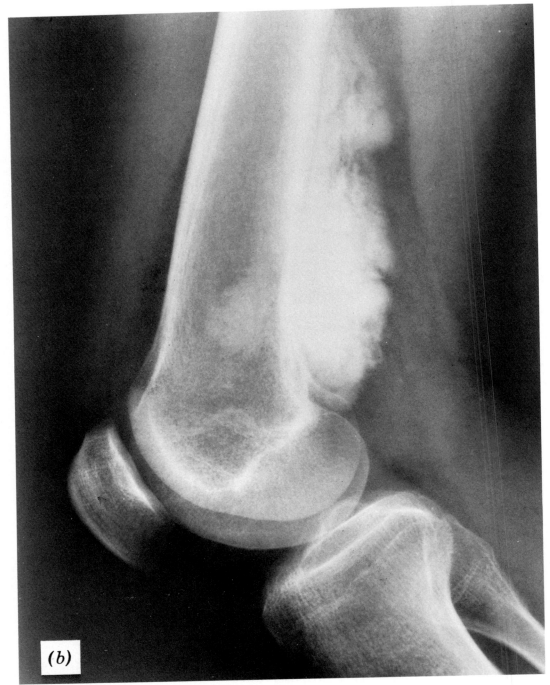

Figure 3.83 (Continued)

CANCERS OF THE HEAD AND NECK

This section includes cancers arising in the oral cavity, oropharynx, nasopharynx, hypopharynx, larynx, paranasal sinuses, nasal fossa, and salivary glands.

INCIDENCE

40,800 projected new cases in the U.S. in 1983
14,250 deaths
4.9% of new cancers in Americans
Male:female ratio 2.7

EPIDEMIOLOGY

Alcohol and tobacco are the major carcinogens for head and neck cancers. Poor oral hygiene, chronic irritation from poorly fitting dentures, and chewing betel nut also play a role. The incidence of adenocarcinomas of the nose and sinus is increased among furniture workers who are exposed to wood dust. There is a marked geographic variation in incidence with very high rates in southeast Asia, southern China, and southern India, where 50% of malignancies in some regions are of head and neck origin. In Chinese patients some association between certain HLA haplotypes and nasopharyngeal cancer exists, and EB virus also appears to be implicated in the same disease. The incidence of head and neck cancers is very low among Mormons, who neither smoke nor drink.

PATHOLOGY

Ninety-five percent of head and neck cancers are squamous cell carcinomas. Adenocarcinomas may arise in the salivary glands, nasopharynx, and nose, while lymphomas can occur in the tonsil and nasopharynx.

Head and neck cancers spread by four modes:

1. Local invasion into muscle, along fascial and muscle planes leading to periosteal invasion and ultimately invasion of bone itself
2. Invasion of the base of skull with perineural tumor extending directly to base of skull, or tumor spread via the parapharyngeal space and then to base of skull with consequent cranial nerve findings

225

3. Lymphatic spread
4. Distant metastasis: relatively uncommon except for pulmonary involvement

SIGNS AND SYMPTOMS

Mass involving neck or face
Oral or nasal bleeding
Pain in face, neck, ear, or throat
Asymptomatic lesion discovered during routine medical or dental examination
Change in speech or hoarse voice
Dysphagia or regurgitation
Weight loss
Trismus
Foul breath
Respiratory distress
Cranial nerve findings
Headache
Cervical adenopathy

DIAGNOSIS AND STAGING

Surgical, needle, or endoscopic biopsy
Meticulous physical examination
Bimanual palpation of oral structures
Direct and indirect laryngoscopy
Computerized tomography of involved region (Figure 3.84)
Contrast laryngography (replaced by CT in most centers)
Lateral soft tissue radiograph or xeroradiograph of the neck (for tumors of hypopharynx and epiglottis)
Cine barium swallow (for tumors of hypopharynx and pyriform sinuses)
Computerized tomography of base of skull to detect local bony invasion or transforaminal extension in patients with cranial nerve symptoms or findings
Chest x-ray films

Because widespread dissemination of head and neck cancer other than to lung is uncommon, routine metastatic evaluation except for chest films is unwarranted unless clinically indicated.

TNM CLASSIFICATION OF HEAD AND NECK CANCERS

T: Primary Tumor

The T classification varies with each site. In some sites (oral cavity, oropharynx, etc.) the T classification depends on tumor size, while in other sites (maxillary sinus, nasopharynx, larynx, etc.) tumor classification depends on tumor extension. The detailed T classification for each site can be found in any textbook of oncology or radiation therapy and will not be listed here.

N: Regional Lymph Nodes (common to all head and neck sites)

NX	Nodes cannot be assessed
N0	No clinically positive node
N1	Single clinically positive homolateral node 3 cm or less in diameter
N2	Single clinically positive homolateral node more than 3 cm but not more than 6 cm in diameter or multiple clinically positive homolateral nodes, none more than 6 cm in diameter
N2a	Single clinically positive homolateral node more than 3 cm but not more than 6 cm in diameter
N2b	Multiple clinically positive homolateral nodes, none more than 6 cm in diameter
N3	Massive homolateral node(s), bilateral nodes, or contralateral node(s)
N3a	Clinically positive homolateral node(s), one more than 6 cm in diameter
N3b	Bilateral clinically positive nodes (in this situation, each side of the neck should be staged separately; that is, N3b, right; N2a, left)
N3c	Contralateral clinically positive node(s) only

M: Distant Metastasis

MX	Not assessed
M0	No (known) distant metastasis
M1	Distant metastasis present

TNM STAGING SYSTEM FOR HEAD AND NECK CANCERS
(common to all head and neck sites)

Stage I	T1 N0 M0
Stage II	T2 N0 M0
Stage III	T3 N0 M0
	T1–3 N1 M0
Stage IV	T4 N0–1 M0
	Any T N2–3 M0
	Any M1

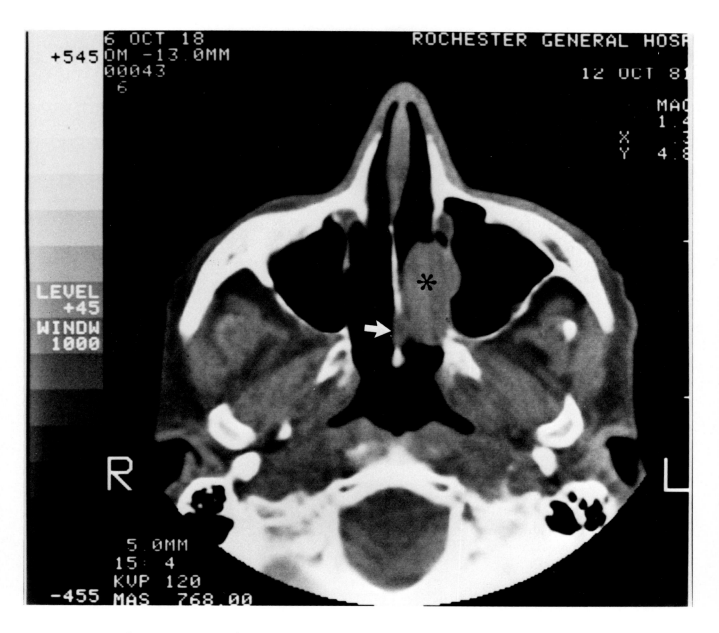

Figure 3.84 *Nasal carcinoma (*) invading the nasal septum (arrow) and medial wall of the left maxillary antrum as seen on this computerized tomogram of the face.*

229

MALIGNANT BRAIN TUMORS

INCIDENCE

12,600 projected new cases in the U.S. in 1983
10,800 deaths
Male:female ratio 1.25
Second most common cause of cancer deaths in children under age 15

EPIDEMIOLOGY

There is some increased incidence of malignant brain tumors among patients with neurofibromatosis, tuberous sclerosis, and Turcot syndrome (familial colonic polyposis and malignant gliomas).

PATHOLOGY

Malignant brain tumors are mainly gliomas, including glioblastoma multiforme, astrocytoma, oligodendroglioma, and ependymoma. Primary sarcomas and lymphomas of brain occur rarely. Metastases to brain from cancers of other primary sites (lung, breast, gastrointestinal tract, kidney, etc.) comprise the most common intracranial malignant process. Confusion with primary brain tumors may arise when the metastasis is solitary.

SIGNS AND SYMPTOMS

Headache
Change in mental function
Emotional lability
Personality alteration
Confusion
Dementia
Seizures
Focal neurologic deficits

DIAGNOSIS AND LOCALIZATION

Computerized tomography (Figure 3.85) has replaced the radionuclide brain scan in most centers

230

Angiography (Figure 3.86); useful for presurgical vascular mapping
Surgical biopsy or excision

Note: In a patient with a known primary extracranial malignancy and multiple metastatic lesions to the brain as seen on CT, a tissue diagnosis of the intracranial lesions is neither necessary nor wise.

EVAUATION FOR METASTASIS

Metastasis of primary brain tumors beyond the central nervous system is extremely rare.

STAGING SYSTEM

There is no TNM or other staging classification of primary brain tumors. Pathologic grade of the tumor has important implications for treatment and prognosis, however.

PATIENT EVALUATION DIAGRAM

See Figure 3.87.

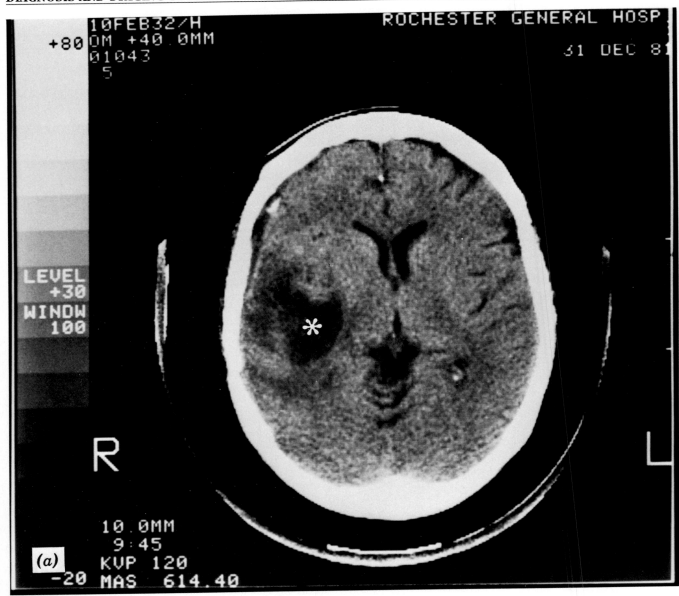

Figure 3.85 (a) Computerized tomogram of the brain without contrast showing a large area of diminished brain density (*) within the right temporal lobe. (b) Following contrast injection, the margins of the lesion (arrows) enhance, which is characteristic but not pathognomonic of primary brain tumors. Surgical biopsy revealed glioblastoma multiforme.

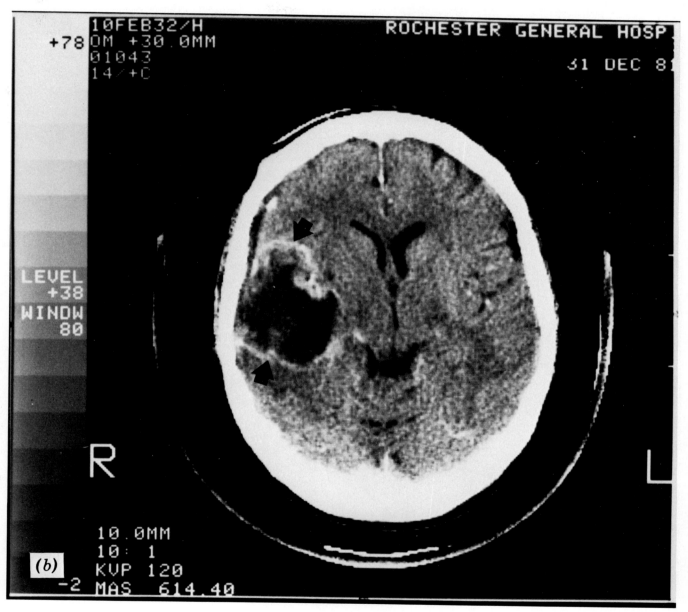

Figure 3.85 (Continued)

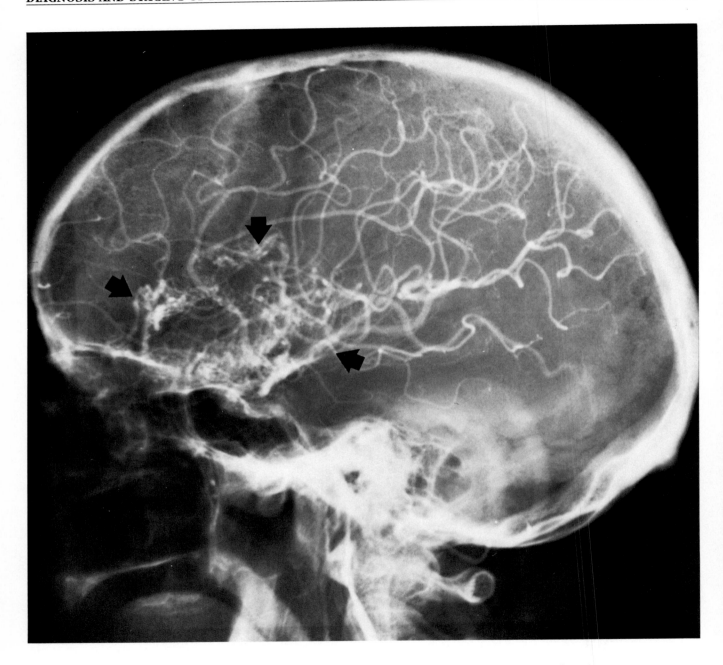

Figure 3.86 *A lateral view from a carotid arteriogram demonstrates the abnormal vascularity (arrows) of a glioma.*

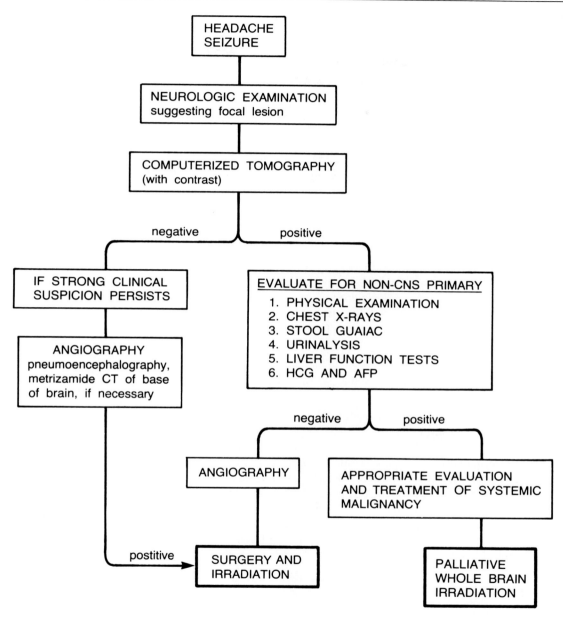

Figure 3.87 *Flow diagram for evaluation of the patient with suspected primary brain tumor. Nearly all malignant brain tumors are visualized with computerized tomography; angiography and other procedures are rarely necessary for diagnostic purposes.*

THYROID CANCER

INCIDENCE

10,200 projected new cases in the U.S. in 1983

1,050 deaths

1.2% of new cancers in Americans

Female:male ratio 2.5

Incidence has been rising in recent years

EPIDEMIOLOGY

Radiation to the head and neck region during childhood is a definite risk factor for thyroid cancer. There is some evidence that patients with endemic goiter have an increased incidence of follicular and anaplastic thyroid cancers. Many medullary carcinomas are familial and occur in association with the Multiple Endocrine Neoplasia syndrome type II (MEN-II).

PATHOLOGY

Papillary carcinoma of the thyroid is the most common type, comprising 60–70% of cases. Follicular carcinoma is next in frequency, representing 20–30% of cases. Only 5–10% are medullary carcinomas, and anaplastic carcinomas are uncommon (1–5%).

Differentiated thyroid cancers—papillary and follicular—tend to be slow-growing, occur in young to middle-aged adults, and usually have long survivals. Medullary carcinomas may secrete various hormones, including calcitonin, prostaglandins, VIP, and ACTH and may occur on a sporadic or a familial basis in the MEN-II syndrome. Anaplastic carcinoma of the thyroid is a highly aggressive, rapidly growing tumor that may distort the contour of the neck and cause obstruction of the airway and esophagus. Survival with this tumor is generally less than one year.

SIGNS AND SYMPTOMS

Asymptomatic thyroid nodule

Hoarse voice

Dysphagia: usually with anaplastic carcinoma

Cervical lymphadenopathy

Symptoms of thyroid hyper- or hypofunction are rare

236

DIAGNOSIS AND STAGING

Careful palpation of the thyroid and cervical and supraclavicular lymph nodes

Radionuclide thyroid scan (Figure 3.88)

Ultrasonography to assess "cold" nodule on thyroid scan

Percutaneous needle aspiration and/or biopsy

Thyroid suppression (with exogenous thyroid hormone) for 3–6 months

Calcitonin levels: medullary carcinoma

Chest x-ray films

Note: In a patient with a previous thyroidectomy for differentiated thyroid cancer:

1. Serum thyroglobulin levels can serve as a marker for residual, recurrent, or metastatic disease.
2. Radioiodine total body scanning may demonstrate pulmonary or osseous metastases if the tumor tissue retains the ability to take up iodine (Figure 3.89).

STAGING SYSTEM

No TNM classification or other staging system for thyroid cancer is in general use.

PATIENT EVALUATION DIAGRAM

See Figure 3.90.

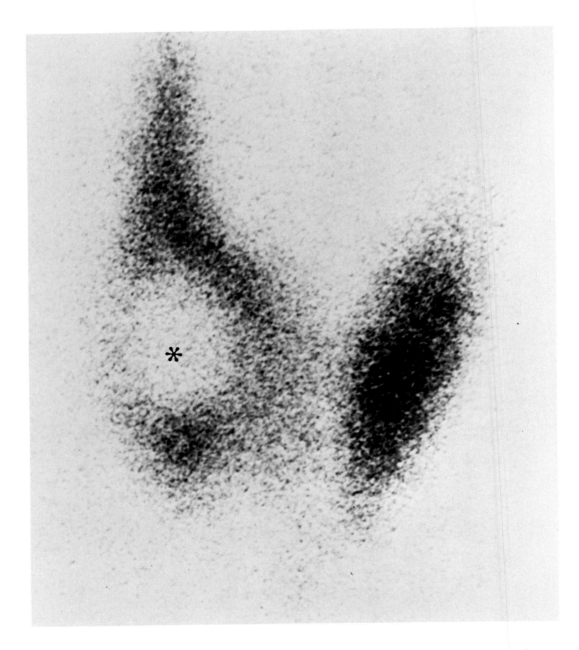

Figure 3.88 Radioisotope scan of the thyroid with a "cold" nodule (*) in the right lobe.

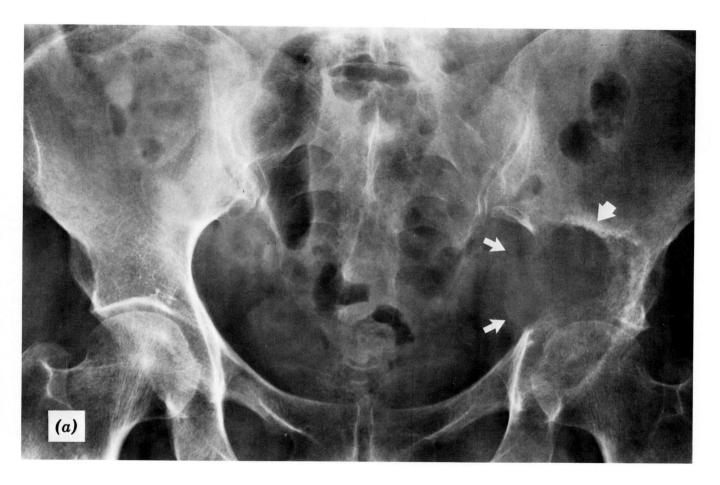

Figure 3.89 (a) Plain film of the pelvis showing an osteolytic metastasis in the left ischium (arrows) in a patient with a previous papillary carcinoma of the thyroid.

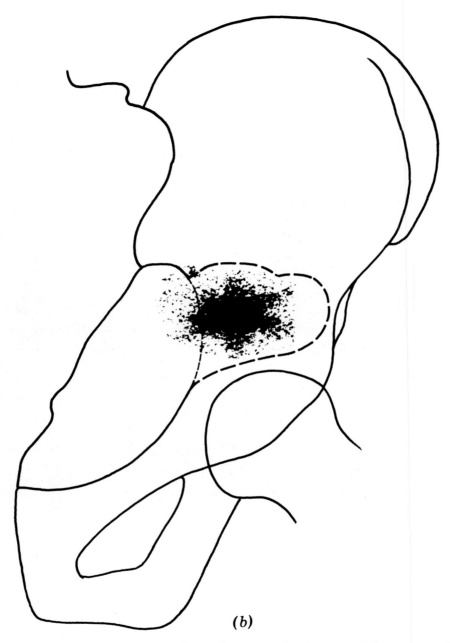

(b)

Figure 3.89 (Continued) (b) ^{131}I *radioisotope body scan of the same patient with superimposed diagram of the left hemipelvis. The area of increased photon activity represents the metastasis. This examination can only be performed in patients who no longer have functioning thyroid glands.*

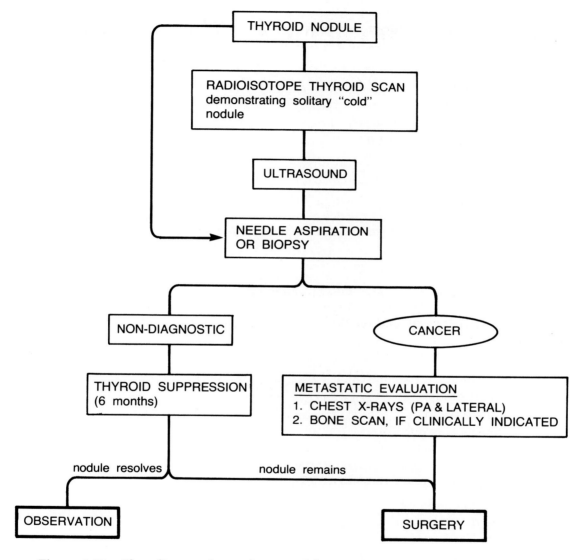

Figure 3.90 *Flow diagram for evaluation of the patient with suspected thyroid cancer.*

241

ADRENOCORTICAL CARCINOMA

INCIDENCE

Approximately two cases per million population in the U.S.
78–132 new cases yearly
Male:female ratio 1.0

PATHOLOGY

It is difficult to diagnose malignancy in an adrenocortical tumor based on histologic criteria alone. Evidence of metastasis is required in order to be certain. Most adrenocortical carcinomas are very large when diagnosed.

SIGNS AND SYMPTOMS

Adrenocortical carcinomas may produce hormones and thus present with characteristic syndromes of hormone excess, or they may be nonfunctioning and present with signs and symptoms related to local invasion or distant metastasis.

Endocrine Syndromes

Cushing's syndrome
Virilization
Feminization
Precocious puberty
Hypoglycemia

Tumor Signs and Symptoms

Abdominal pain
Abdominal mass
Weight loss
Anorexia
Fever, malaise

DIAGNOSIS

The diagnosis of adrenocortical carcinoma depends on recognition of the endocrine manifestations and demonstration of an adrenal mass. Exploratory laparotomy is usually necessary to establish a tissue diagnosis and determine resectability.

Measurement of steroid hormone plasma levels and urinary metabolites

Suppression tests of relevant steroid hormones

Computerized tomography to detect adrenal mass and assess local extension and hepatic metastases

Ultrasonography (Figure 3.91); useful to distinguish between renal and extrarenal origin of tumor

^{131}I-19-iodocholesterol or 6-^{131}I-iodomethyl-19-norcholesterol radionuclide scan; useful for functioning adrenal tumors

Arteriography (Figure 3.92) for presurgical vascular mapping

STAGING SYSTEM

A TNM classification is not available for adrenocortical carcinoma. A useful staging system is given below.

Stage I   Tumor <5 cm, negative nodes, no local invasion, no metastases
Stage II   Tumor >5 cm, negative nodes, no local invasion, no metastases
Stage III   Positive nodes or local invasion
Stage IV   Positive nodes and local invasion or distant metastases

PATIENT EVALUATION DIAGRAM

See Figure 3.93.

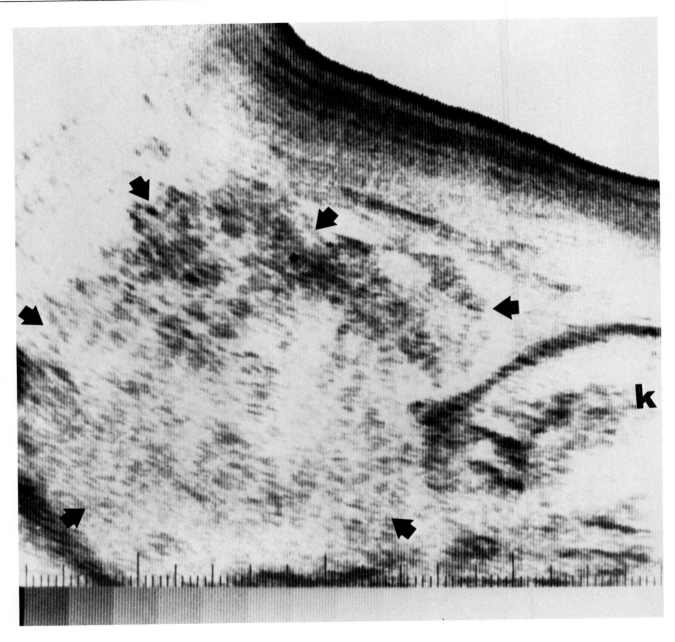

Figure 3.91 Longitudinal ultrasound through the right upper quadrant of a patient with back pain and a flank mass. A large tumor (arrows) is seen superior to the kidney (k). At surgery an adrenocortical carcinoma was found.

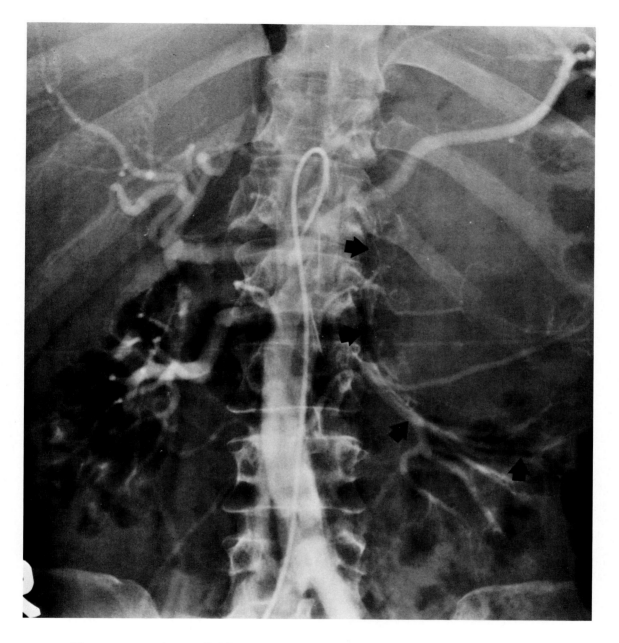

Figure 3.92 Aortic flush angiogram demonstrating a large left suprarenal tumor (arrows). Note the hypovascularity of the tumor mass. The angiogram is not diagnostic of an adrenal carcinoma; however, the study does verify the presence of a tumor, and subsequent surgery confirmed its suspected adrenal origin.

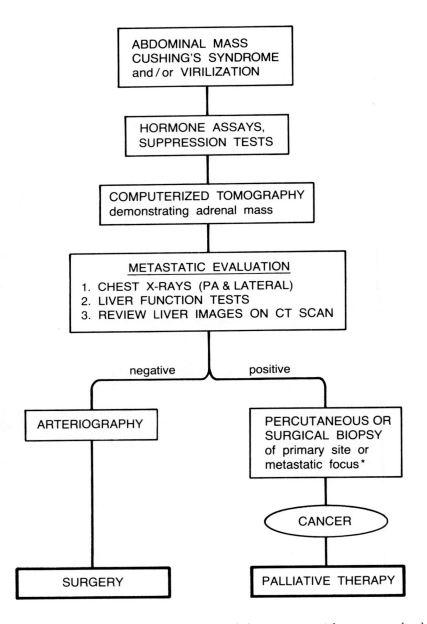

Figure 3.93 *Flow digram for evaluation of the patient with suspected adrenocortical carcinoma. * The purpose of the biopsy is to establish a tissue diagnosis of malignancy and confirm its adrenal origin, if possible.*

ISLET CELL CARCINOMAS OF THE PANCREAS

INCIDENCE

Approximately one case per 100,000 population in the U.S.
190–250 new cases yearly
Male:female ratio 1.0

EPIDEMIOLOGY

Many cases are familial and are associated with the Multiple Endocrine Neoplasia syndrome. Peak incidence occurs between ages 40 and 70, but the tumors may arise at any age.

PATHOLOGY

Islet cell tumors may be found in as many as 1.5% of carefully performed autopsies, but most are benign. Malignancy in islet cell carcinomas is difficult to diagnose on histologic grounds alone; evidence of metastatic disease is required for a definite determination. Islet cell carcinomas are frequently multiple and often quite small (<2 cm).

SIGNS AND SYMPTOMS

Tumor Type	Hormone	Clinical Syndrome
Insulinoma	Insulin	Hypoglycemia
Gastrinoma (Zollinger–Ellison syndrome)	Gastrin	Peptic ulcer, diarrhea
Glucagonoma	Glucagon	Diabetes, skin rash (necrolytic migratory erythema), weight loss, stomatitis
Pancreatic cholera	Vasoactive intestinal polypeptide (VIP), possibly other hormones	Watery diarrhea, hypokalemia, achlorhydria
Somatostatinoma	Somatostatin	Cholelithiasis, diabetes, steatorrhea
PPoma	Pancreatic polypeptide	?

DIAGNOSIS

Assay of the relevant hormone, with use of provocative tests in some cases

Computerized tomography (1) of the pancreas, employing high detail, thin section technique; (2) of the liver, using regular technique, to detect liver metastases

Superselective pancreatic arteriography (Figure 3.94)

Pancreatic venous sampling for hormone levels; may be useful if radiologic methods do not localize the tumor

Exploratory surgery: usually required for tissue diagnosis

STAGING SYSTEM

No TNM classification or other staging system is available for islet cell carcinomas.

PATIENT EVALUATION DIAGRAM

See Figure 3.95.

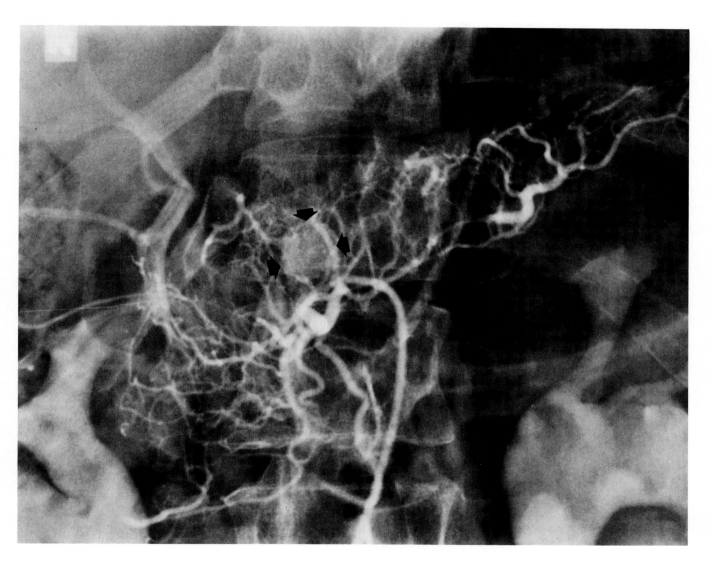

Figure 3.94 Magnified superselective pancreatic angiogram documenting the presence of a 2-cm islet cell tumor (arrows). Previous ultrasound and thin section, high detail computerized tomography failed to identify the lesion.

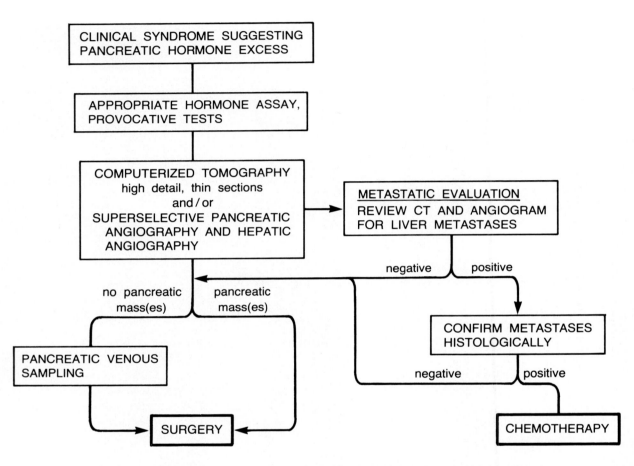

Figure 3.95 *Flow diagram for evaluation of the patient with suspected islet cell carcinoma of the pancreas. Note: The management of gastrinoma is controversial and undergoing considerable evolution. Therefore, this schema may not strictly apply to this tumor.*

CHAPTER 4

Evaluation of Patients with Cancer of Unknown Origin

Metastatic cancer presenting without a known primary malignancy is a common problem, comprising 5–10% of most oncology practices. Such cases may present with malignant hepatomegaly (Figure 4.1), pleural effusion, or metastases to lung, bone, brain, lymph nodes, skin, or other sites. The first step in the evaluation of such a patient is a meticulous history and physical examination. Frequently overlooked points include (1) a history of a pigmented skin lesion removed in the past; (2) biopsy or excision of a "benign" tumor in the past; (3) a history of vaginal bleeding in a postmenopausal woman; (4) a thorough examination of the skin including subungual areas; (5) pelvic and rectal examinations; and (6) ear, nose, and throat examination.

A careful review of the pathologic material with the pathologist is critical. If, for example, the pathologic diagnosis is lymphoma or melanoma, no further search for a primary tumor is necessary. A squamous histology suggests an origin in the uterine cervix, upper aerodigestive tract, or lung, directing the diagnostic work-up to a pelvic exam, an ENT exam, an esophagram, and a chest x-ray.

Most metastases of unknown primary origin are adenocarcinomas, with a very wide spectrum of possible sites of origin. Often the pathologist can offer morphologic clues to the tissue of tumor origin. In other cases such hints are not available, and the physician must then decide how extensive the search for a primary site should be, bearing in mind that the disease is already disseminated and that discovery of the primary would not have any implications for cure.

251

The only reason for seeking the primary site of origin is to determine the most effective form of systemic therapy. Certain adenocarcinomas, especially those of breast, thyroid, ovarian, and prostatic origin, are particularly amenable to specific types of systemic therapy. For example, knowing that a painful bone metastasis derives from an occult primary breast cancer has important implications for treatment and prognosis. On the other hand, knowing that extensive liver metastases derive from an occult lesion in the cecum, the pancreas, or the gall bladder has little therapeutic significance, since no effective systemic therapy exists for any of these problems. For these reasons the evaluation of a patient presenting with metastatic adenocarcinoma of unknown primary origin should be directed toward detection of treatable malignancies.

In women the evaluation should include careful physical examination of the breasts, the thyroid, and the pelvis and limited but appropriate imaging, including bilateral mammography, thyroid scan, and ultrasound of the pelvis. In men digital rectal examination with careful palpation of the prostate is required. If the clinical picture is suggestive (i.e., blastic bone metastases), blind needle biopsy of the prostate is appropriate if a palpable nodule is not detected.

In most cases if gastrointestinal symptoms are absent, stool guaiacs are negative, and hemoglobin level is normal, radiographic and endoscopic studies of the gastrointestinal tract are not productive, and the chance discovery of an occult lesion would not influence subsequent management. Similarly, if pulmonary symptoms are absent and the routine chest film is negative, no therapeutic advantage is gained by computerized or plain film tomography of the chest to detect an occult primary lung cancer.

In a majority of cases of adenocarcinoma of unknown primary origin, the primary site is never detected, even at postmortem examination. Such primaries may have undergone spontaneous regression or may simply be too small to be found by any means. Rather than embark on a costly, sometimes risky, and ultimately futile diagnostic crusade, the physician should plan a limited and thoughtful investigation directed at identifying treatable malignancies and then tailor therapy to the clinical situation. Such a policy will minimize patient risk, discomfort, and expense without affecting the ultimate prognosis.

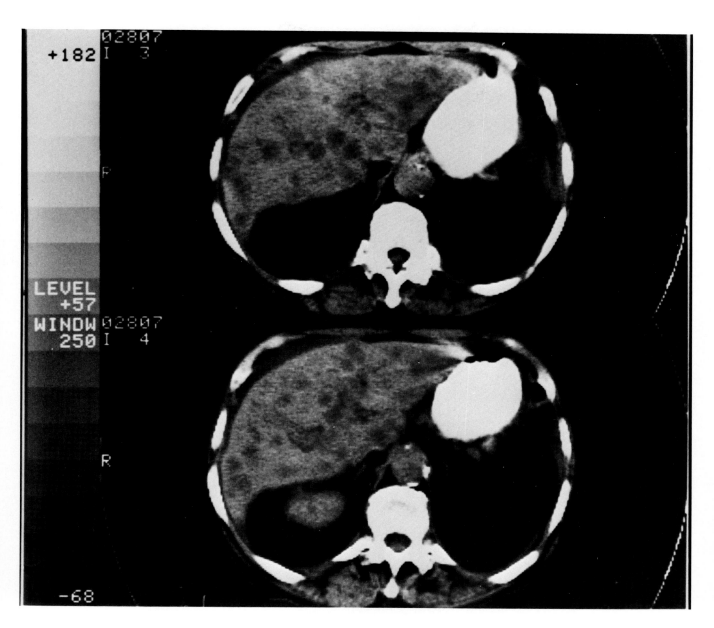

Figure 4.1 CT scan showing hepatic metastases, which were the presenting manifestation in a patient with adenocarcinoma of unknown origin.

CHAPTER 5

Oncologic Emergencies: Diagnostic Evaluation

Cancer patients are subject to a variety of acute complications caused either by their underlying malignant disease or by its therapy. The ability of cancers to obstruct blood vessels, ureters, and other structures, to produce ectopic hormones or to release cellular products, and the effects of treatment in altering host defenses and bone marrow function all combine to make cancer patients prone to serious emergency events. With recent developments in cancer treatment resulting in improved survival for many patients, prompt recognition and appropriate treatment of oncologic emergencies takes on an increased importance.

Discussed below are several emergency problems encountered frequently among cancer patients that require various imaging modalities for diagnosis and elucidation. Purely medical problems such as thrombocytopenic hemorrhage, sepsis, and tumor lysis syndrome are outside the scope of this text and will not be discussed.

SUPERIOR VENA CAVA SYNDROME

SIGNS AND SYMPTOMS

Signs and symptoms of superior vena cava syndrome include edema of the face, neck, and upper extremities; cyanosis of the face and neck; prominent venous pattern over the chest; hoarseness; stridor; chest pain; dyspnea; cough; and neck vein distention.

PATHOPHYSIOLOGY

Superior vena cava syndrome is caused by extrinsic compression of the superior vena cava and its tributaries and/or by thrombosis of the superior vena cava due to a mass in the superior mediastinum. The superior vena cava is thin-walled and has a low intravascular pressure so that it is easily compressed. Also, it is located within a rigid, nondistensible compartment, which makes vascular compression more likely.

ETIOLOGY

Approximately 80% of cases are due to malignancies, most commonly lung cancer, lymphomas, and breast cancer. Benign causes include thrombosis due to central venous catheters, pericardial disease, dermoid cyst, histoplasmosis, and others.

DIAGNOSIS

The chest x-ray film reveals a mediastinal mass in almost every case associated with malignancy (Figure 5.1). The radionuclide superior vena cavagram (Figure 5.2) confirms the diagnosis and demonstrates the obstruction and resulting collateral circulation. Iodinated contrast superior vena cavography is rarely required. Tissue diagnosis, in a patient without a prior diagnosis of malignancy, is usually made by bronchoscopy, sputum cytology, lymph node biopsy, or thoracotomy.

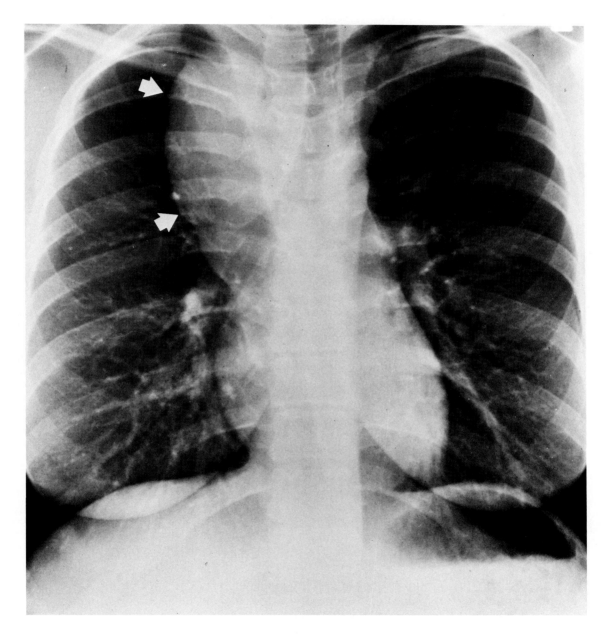

Figure 5.1 Large mediastinal mass (arrows) in a patient with nodular sclerosing Hodgkin's disease and signs of superior vena caval obstruction.

257

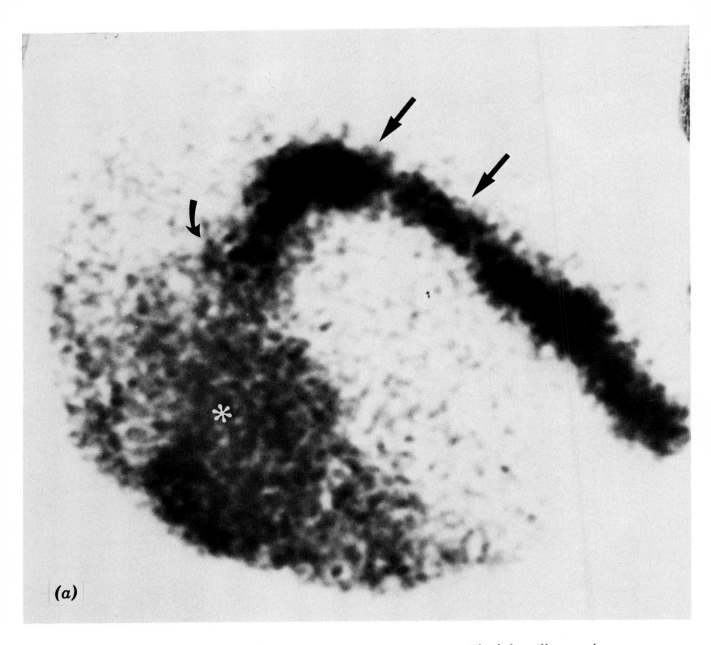

Figure 5.2 (a) Normal isotope superior vena cavagram. The left axillary and subclavian veins (straight arrows) empty into a nonobstructed superior vena cava (curved arrow) and ultimately into the heart (*). (b) Obstructed superior vena cava manifested by collateral flow into the internal mammary (long curved arrows) and intercostal (sharply curved arrows) veins. The axillary and subclavian veins are seen (long arrows), but cardiac filling has not occurred.

258

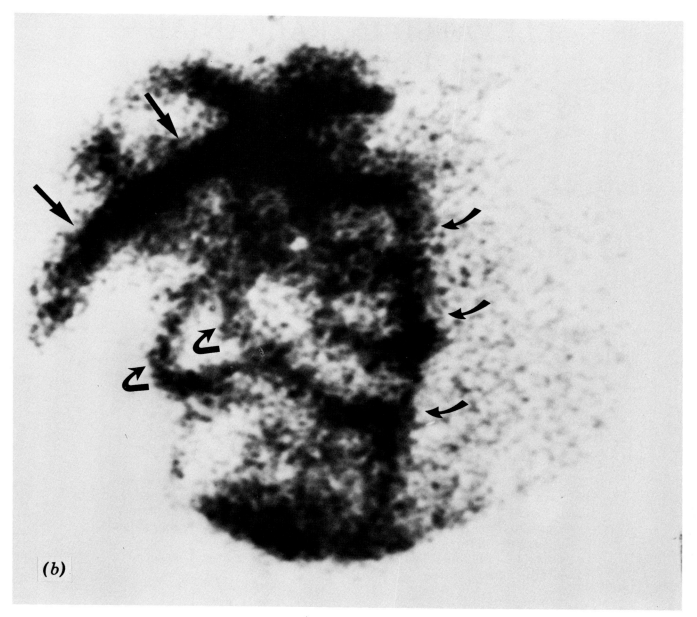

Figure 5.2 (Continued)

ELEVATED INTRACRANIAL PRESSURE

SIGNS AND SYMPTOMS

Early symptoms may include personality change, headache, visual blurring, nausea, vomiting, and decreased level of consciousness. Physical signs include papilledema, emotional lability, confusion, dementia, and focal neurologic findings involving motor or sensory function, speech, or cranial nerves. Seizures may occur.

PATHOPHYSIOLOGY

Focal effects of brain tumors may be irritative, causing seizures, or destructive, causing focal deficits. Increased intracranial pressure is partially produced by tumor mass and partially by the surrounding edema. Metastatic tumors often produce cerebral edema out of proportion to their size.

ETIOLOGY

Elevated intracranial pressure in cancer patients is most often caused by metastases to the brain (usually from cancers of the lung, breast, kidney, gastrointestinal tract, and melanoma), but may also arise in patients with primary brain tumors and in those with meningeal infiltration with leukemias, lymphomas, and occasionally solid tumors.

DIAGNOSIS

The diagnosis depends primarily on recognition of suspicious findings on history and thorough neurologic evaluation. Computerized tomography of the head (Figure 5.3), with contrast enhancement, is the imaging procedure of choice and has rendered skull films, radionuclide brain scanning, pneumoencephalography, and angiography obsolete and unnecessary in this setting. Lumbar puncture with spinal fluid analysis including cytology will detect most cases of meningeal tumor.

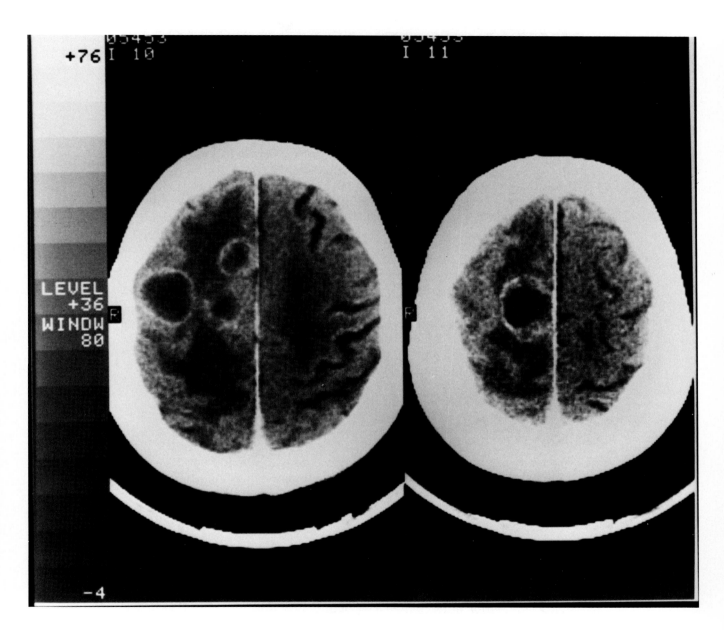

Figure 5.3 CT scan showing multiple cerebral metastases in a patient with metastatic malignant melanoma.

261

SPINAL CORD COMPRESSION

SIGNS AND SYMPTOMS

Back pain is almost invariably the earliest and most prominent symptom. It is constant and may be exacerbated by movement, coughing, or sneezing or by neck flexion and straight leg raising. The pain may have a radicular component. Numbness, tingling, sensory loss, paraplegia, urinary hesitancy with eventual retention and overflow, and constipation also occur. Physical findings include tenderness at the level of vertebral involvement, depression of appropriate deep tendon reflexes, motor weakness, and hypesthesia or dysesthesia in the involved dermatome. A sensory level is usually present and in most cases is a good indicator of the site of the lesion to within one or two vertebral bodies.

PATHOPHYSIOLOGY

Metastatic tumor extending from vertebral bodies to the epidural space is the most common mechanism. The neurologic deficit may be due to direct compression of the spinal cord (or cauda equina) by the epidural tumor, to ischemia secondary to involvement by tumor of the blood supply to the cord, or to vertebral compression or collapse due to pathologic fracture. Invasion of the spinal cord itself by extension through the dura is rare. Intramedullary metastasis, although rare, may produce a clinical picture indistinguishable from that of cord compression.

ETIOLOGY

The frequency of tumor types responsible for cord compression parallels their tendency to involve bone. Cancers of the lung, breast, lymphomas, myeloma, and prostate are most common, but almost any malignancy may produce this problem.

DIAGNOSIS

The diagnosis depends on a high index of suspicion, recognition of the clinical picture, and demonstration of vertebral involvement by plain films (Figure 5.4) or bone scan (positive in more than 85% of patients). Myelography (Figure 5.5) reveals a complete block to the passage of contrast in 75% of cases and a high grade partial block in 25%. The block is located at the site of vertebral bony involvement in 85% of cases.

Computerized tomographic scanning of the spine (Figure 5.6) with or without intrathecal metrizamide has recently become the imaging modality of choice for spinal cord compression in many centers. Unlike conventional contrast myelography, which demonstrates only an impression on the dura, CT of the spine actually visualizes the tumor in the adjacent vertebral body and spinal canal and provides a more direct method of diagnosis.

Spinal fluid analysis is helpful in detecting meningeal spread of tumor. Spinal fluid protein is almost invariably elevated in cases of cord compression.

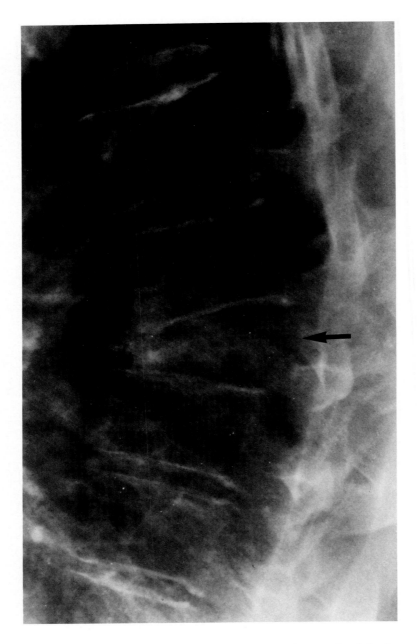

Figure 5.4 *Lateral film of the thoracic spine with vertebral body collapse (arrows).*

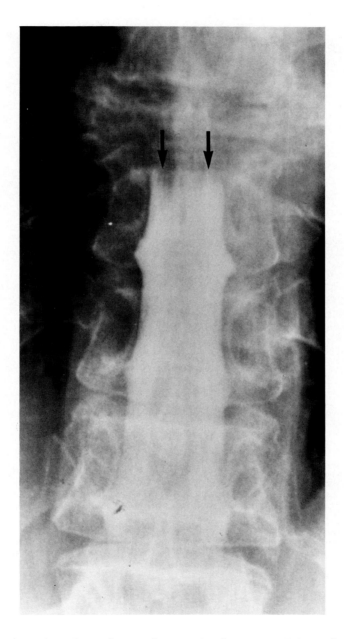

Figure 5.5   Anterior view of a myelogram in the same patient showing complete obstruction (arrows) at the level of vertebral collapse.

265

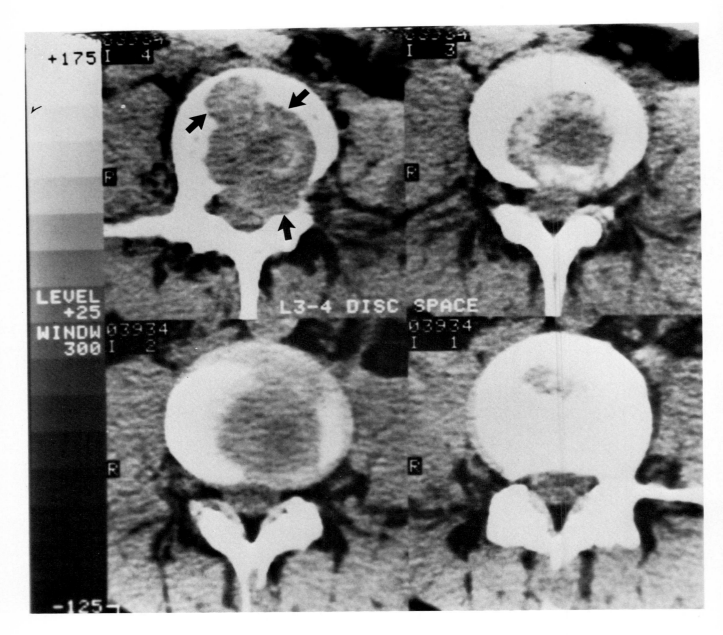

Figure 5.6 Computerized tomographic sections of a vertebral body showing metastatic tumor involving the bone and extending into the spinal canal (arrows).

CARDIAC TAMPONADE

SIGNS AND SYMPTOMS

Cardiac tamponade produces chest pain, anxiety, dyspnea, cough, hypotension, pallor, diaphoresis, neck vein engorgement, decreased pulse pressure, pulsus paradoxus, and distant heart sounds. Pericardial friction rub and arrhythmias are often present as well.

PATHOPHYSIOLOGY

The severity of neoplastic cardiac tamponade depends on the rate of accumulation of pericardial fluid, the amount of fluid, and the distensibility of the pericardium. Because the pericardium is frequently involved with tumor and hence less distensible, neoplastic tamponade may occur more rapidly than benign tamponade.

ETIOLOGY

Cancers of the lung and breast, leukemias and lymphomas, melanomas, sarcomas, and gastrointestinal cancers are most frequently responsible for malignant pericardial disease.

DIAGNOSIS

Physical examination should suggest the diagnosis. Chest x-ray films often show an enlarged heart, but a normal chest x-ray film does not exclude the possibility of tamponade. The EKG (Figure 5.7) may show total electrical alternans (involving atrial and ventricular complexes), which is almost pathognomonic of cardiac tamponade. Cardiac ultrasonography (Figure 5.8) is the quickest, safest, and most reliable means to detect pericardial effusion and may suggest the presence of tamponade as well.

Emergency pericardiocentesis may be necessary before an ultrasound can be obtained in cases where the diagnosis seems highly likely and the situation seems life-threatening. The pericardial fluid removed should always be sent for cytologic examination.

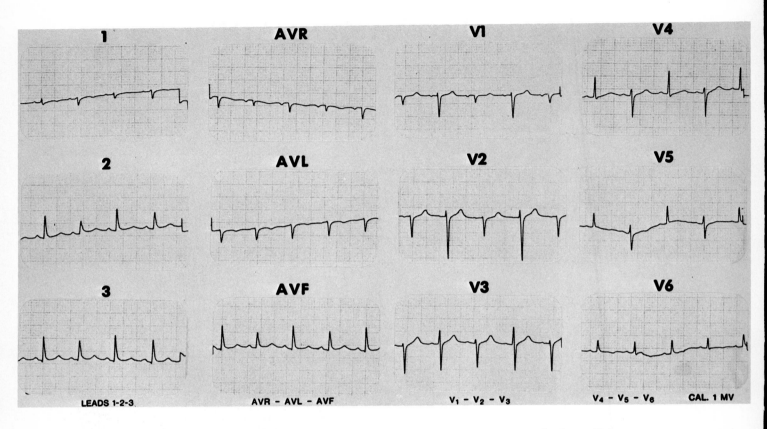

Figure 5.7 EKG demonstrating electrical alternans seen particularly well in leads 2, V_1, V_2, V_4, and V_5.

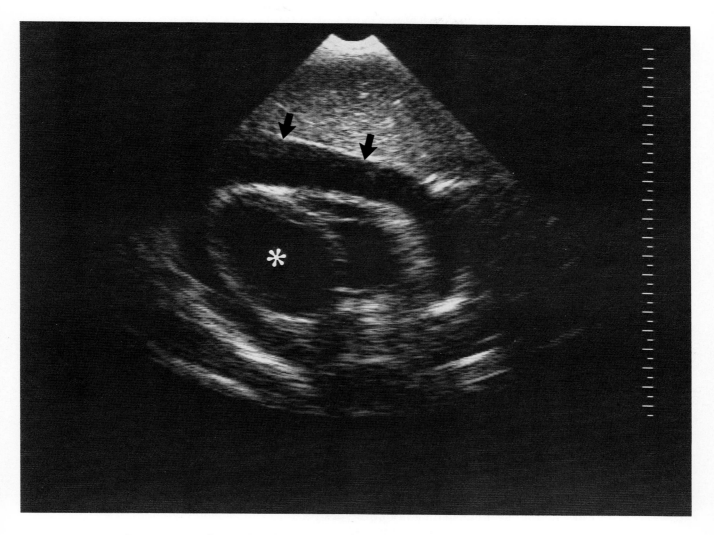

Figure 5.8 *Echocardiogram of a patient with tamponade. The effusion is seen anterior to the heart (arrows). The left ventricle is marked (*). (Courtesy of Dr. Laura vonDoenhoff.)*

269

BILATERAL URETERAL OBSTRUCTION

SIGNS AND SYMPTOMS

Symptoms vary with the degree of uremia, but abdominal or back pain and oliguria or anuria are almost invariable. Nausea, vomiting, lethargy, confusion, and other uremic symptoms are progressive. An abdominal or pelvic mass may be present on physical examination.

PATHOPHYSIOLOGY

While metastases to the ureters rarely occur, most cases of ureteral obstruction are caused by extrinsic compression or direct invasion of the ureters by retroperitoneal or pelvic malignancies. Obstruction may occur at any level of the ureter.

ETIOLOGY

Extensive retroperitoneal adenopathy or large pelvic mass secondary to carcinomas of the cervix, ovary, colon, prostate, bladder, and the malignant lymphomas may produce bilateral ureteral obstruction and consequent renal failure. The resulting uremia may develop insidiously and occasionally may be the presenting symptom of a hitherto unrecognized malignancy.

DIAGNOSIS

The development of oliguric or anuric renal failure in a patient with cancer should raise the possibility of bilateral ureteral obstruction. Computerized tomography (without contrast) provides confirmation of the diagnosis and may indicate the level and the nature of the obstruction. Ultrasonography and radionuclide renal scanning are alternative procedures for demonstrating obstruction, but these modalities do not yield other useful information usually available from CT scanning. If percutaneous (or surgical) nephrostomies are placed for therapeutic purposes, contrast nephrostograms may be performed to define the exact site of obstruction.

Suggestions for Additional Reading

Devita VT, Hellman S, Rosenberg SA, eds. *Cancer: Principles and Practice of Oncology.* Philadelphia: JB Lippincott, 1982.

Haskell CM, ed. *Cancer Treatment.* Philadelphia: WB Saunders, 1980.

Holland JF, Frei E, eds. *Cancer Medicine.* Philadelphia: Lea & Febiger, 1982.

Rosenthal SN, Bennett JM, eds. *Practical Cancer Chemotherapy.* Garden City: Medical Examination, 1981.

Steckel RJ, Kagan RA, eds. *Diagnosis and Staging of Cancer: A Radiologic Approach.* Philadelphia: WB Saunders, 1976.

Steckel RJ, Kagan RA, eds. *Cancer Diagnosis: New Concepts and Techniques.* New York: Grune & Stratton, 1982.

Willis, RA: *The Spread of Tumors in the Human Body.* London: Butterworth, 1973.

Yarbro JW, Bornstein RS, eds. *Oncologic Emergencies.* New York: Grune & Stratton, 1981.